PHARMACOLOGY from A to Z

CW00558677

Pharmacology from **A** to **Z**

John Carpenter

Lecture in Pharmacology, University of Manchester

Manchester University Press **መ**

Manchester and New York

Distributed exclusively in the USA and Canada
by St. Martin's Press

Copyright © John Carpenter 1988

Published by Manchester University Press
Oxford Road, Manchester M13 9PL, UK
and Room 400, 175 Fifth Avenue, New York, NY 10100, USA

Distributed exclusively in the USA and Canada
by St. Martin's Press, Inc.,
175 Fifth Avenue, New York, NY 10100, USA

British Library cataloguing in publication data
Carpenter, John
　　Pharmacology from A to Z.
　　1. Drugs – Encyclopaedias
　　I. Title
　　615'.1'0321

Library of Congress cataloging in publication data
Carpenter, John, 1943–
　　Pharmacology from A to Z / John Carpenter
　　p. cm. ISBN 0-7190-2988-0 : $35.00 (U.S. : est.). ISBN 0-7190-2692 (pbk.) :
　　$15.00 (U.S. : est.). 1. Pharmacology—Outlines, syllabi, etc. 2. Drugs—Dictionaries.
　　I. Title.
　　　　[DNLM: 1. Drugs.　　QV 55 Cd295p]
　　RM301.14.C37 1988
　　615'.1.–dc19
　　DNLM/DLC

ISBN 0 7190 2988 0 *hardback*
ISBN 0 7190 2692 X *paperback*

Typeset by Koinonia Ltd, Manchester
Printed in Great Britain
by Hartnolls Ltd, Bodmin, Cornwall

CONTENTS

Preface — *page* vii
Introduction — viii
How to use this book — ix
Abbreviations — x

Pharmacology from A to Z — 1

Rapid reference — 111

PREFACE

Many students find when they begin to study Pharmacology for the first time that the subject seems to require that they learn an enormous number of seemingly unrelated facts. After a period of time many find that connections begin to appear between these facts, although for too many students, the experience is that many of the facts they have learned to pass their examinations remain firmly unconnected to anything at all. This could either be because the connections have not yet been made, or that the facts are indeed isolated from the rest of the discipline. In this case, it could well be argued that these particular items of information are worthless. The purpose of this little book is to make it easier for you (the student) to distinguish the essentials of Pharmacology from the details – to tell the wood from the trees, if you like. If the objectives of this book are met, you will begin to grasp the important central concepts about drugs more easily – you might then find that some of those facts are in fact not quite so isolated and some will prove to be so fascinating that you will develop a burning urge to find out why those particular drugs have those unusual properties. When that happens you will have taken the first step towards becoming a pharmacologist.

Into *Pharmacology from A to Z* has been distilled, not the wisdom of 20 years of undergraduates, but their problems, for this is a book for the average and below average student – if you are a high flier, you may find it gives you a useful start, but you will soon be immersed in thick textbooks with copious references – well before the average undergraduate has mastered this A-Z!

If you like this book, please let me know. If it irritates you or you believe it can be improved, please also let me know how and I will do my best to incorporate your suggestions into any revised impressions that are are made.

John Carpenter
January 1988

INTRODUCTION

The book is arranged in two parts; an alphabetical listing of drugs and their properties forms the first of these and a rapid reference section, in which the drugs are arranged in groups according to a simple classification system, forms the second – what might be referred to as an "anti-index".

There are essentially three types of drug included in this book. Firstly there are those that are typical of all the drugs in that group – these are the prototypes and are given a full entry in the alphabetical section and appear in **CAPITALS** in the **RAPID REFERENCE** section. Secondly, there are other members of these groups which are to all intents and purposes identical to the prototypes in their main properties. These are not given full entries in the alphabetical section, but are described simply as being "As **PROTOTYPE**", although important differences are summarised. The third group comprises those drugs which are not much like anything else and are not important enough to be included in the beginner student's core of essential information. They are there to amuse, to interest and to stimulate.

HOW TO USE THIS BOOK

It is assumed that you already have another, primary textbook of Pharmacology and that you will be attending lectures from which you will be producing your own notes. What is intended is that you use the alphabetical section of this book to look up all the drugs mentioned in your lectures. This will summarise for you the important properties of these drugs. What you will not find is a list of the effects these drugs produce. To determine the effects drugs produce you will need to refer to your Pharmacology textbook and your lecture notes. You will also need to consult your textbooks and notes for the foundation subjects, such as Physiology, Biochemistry, Chemistry, etc. What should emerge is a framework of the essential properties of drugs and a central core to which you can keep referring in order to deduce the effects of particular drugs.

When the time comes for you to revise for your examinations, you can use the **RAPID REFERENCE** section. You will be able to see at a glance those drugs that are worth studying in detail (**PROTOTYPES**) and those that are worth only glancing at because they have the same profile as the **PROTOTYPES**. You should also be able to identify those drugs that are really such "small print" as to require an electron microscope!

You will probably find that my selection of **PROTOTYPES** does not coincide exactly with that of your lecturers. In this case, make the necessary annotations to the **RAPID REFERENCE** section yourself. (The basis on which the **PROTOTYPES** have been chosen is that they are usually those described in the *British National Formulary* (BNF) as being the most appropriate therapeutically. For drugs that have no therapeutic value but are of interest from a theoretical point of view, I have used my own judgement wherever I have not been able to find a consensus opinion in the commoner Pharmacology textbooks. I have relied quite heavily upon *Basic Pharmacology*, edited by R. W. Foster and published by Butterworths).

The naming of drugs is always a thorny issue. Throughout this book, *British Pharmacopœia* (BP) approved names are used, although a few common *United States Pharmacopeia* (USP) names are listed in the alphabetic section, though without full entries. For these USP names, cross references are given to the appropriate BP name. Trade names are avoided.

ABBREVIATIONS

Some abbreviations (e.g. ACTH) are listed as alphabetic entries. However, some are not and these are listed and defined below:–

ACE	Angiotensin converting enzyme
ACh	Acetylcholine
AChE	Acetylcholinesterase (true cholinesterase)
BNF	*British National Formulary*
BP	*British Pharmacopœia*
ChE	Butyrylcholinesterase (cholinesterase, pseudo-cholinesterase)
COMT	Catechol-O-methyl transferase
CNS	Central nervous system
CSF	Cerebrospinal fluid
CTZ	Chemosensitive trigger zone
DHF	Dihydrofolate
GI	Gastro-intestinal
IgE	Immunoglubulin type E
MAO	Monoamine oxidase
MFO	Mixed function oxidase
OTC	Over the counter, i.e. without prescription
PG	Prostaglandin
POM	Prescription only medicine
SER	Smooth endoplasmic reticulum
USP	*United States Pharmacopeia*

ACEBUTALOL

As **PROPRANOLOL** but some cardioselectivity (β_1–adrenoceptors) and some intrinsic activity.

ACENOCOUMAROL

See **NICOUMAROL**.

ACETAMINOPHEN (USP)

See **PARACETAMOL**.

ACETANALID

As **ASPIRIN**, but too toxic for use in man.

ACETAZOLAMIDE

Carbonic anhydrase inhibitor.

Uses:– i) glaucoma
ii) may be of use in epilepsy (Grand Mal & Focal seizures; cf. ketogenic diet).

Precautions:– adverse effects common, especially in the elderly; augments K^+ excretion and may cause depression.

ACETOHEXIMIDE

As **TOLBUTAMIDE** but longer half-life (approximately 45 h including active metabolites).

ACETYLCHOLINE

Agonist at muscarinic and nicotinic cholinoceptors (normal transmitter in cholinergic neurones).

Readily hydrolysed, spontaneously or enzymically. Substrate for:–
i) acetylcholinesterase (true cholinesterase; AChE) at cholinergic neuro-effector junctions and in erythrocytes
ii) butyrylcholinesterase (cholinesterase; pseudocholinesterase; ChE) in solution in plasma and in liver.

Uses:– as experimental tool.

See also:– bethanechol, carbachol, DMPP, furtrethonium, methacholine, muscarine, nicotine, oxotremorine, pilocarpine, suxamethonium.

ACETYLCYSTEINE

Replenishes hepatic stores of glutathione depleted by overdoses of **PARACETAMOL**. Also lowers viscosity of mucus by breaking disulphide bonds.

Uses:– i) treatment of overdosing with **PARACETAMOL**.

ii) as aerosol to help respiration by facilitating expectoration – benefit unsubstantiated.

2-(ACETOXY)-BENZOIC ACID

See **ASPIRIN**.

ACETYLSALICYLIC ACID

See **ASPIRIN**.

ACETYLTRIETHYLCHOLINE

False transmitter in cholinergic nerves. Structural analogue of **ACETYL-CHOLINE**. Much less potent at cholinoceptors than **ACETYL-CHOLINE**.

Formed in cholinergic nerves by acetylation of **TRIETHYL-CHOLINE**

ACONITINE

Delays inactivation of Na^+ channels – hence repetitive firing and failure of transmission.

Naturally occurring in the common aconite or monkshood (*Aconitum napellus*).

Uses:– i) experimental tool.

ii) at one time used as tincture to relieve inflammatory pain.

See also:– batrachotoxin, dicophane, pyrethrin, veratridine.

ACTH (ADRENOCORTICOTROPHIC HORMONE; CORTICOTROPHIN)

Trophic hormone released from the anterior pituitary in response to low circulating levels of adrenocorticosteroids. Effect is to stimulate production of adrenocorticosteroids – mainly **CORTICOSTERONE** and **HYDRO-CORTISONE**.

Polypeptide with 39 residues.

See also:– tetracosactrin.

ACTINOMYCIN D

Cytotoxic antibiotic – inhibits transcription (mRNA synthesis) by binding in minor groove of DNA.

Poorly lipid soluble – hence must be injected.

Uses:– i) to treat paediatric cancers esp. rhabdomyosarcoma and Wilm's tumour.

ii) as experimental tool – inhibits protein synthesis at very early stage.

Precautions:– damages all rapidly dividing cell types.

See also:– bleomycin, cycloheximide, doxorubicin.

ACYCLOVIR

Anti-viral agent (herpes). Metabolised in infected cells to acyclo-GTP which inhibits viral polymerase. Also incorporated into viral DNA; transcription stops when this modified base encountered.

Uses:– i) treatment of herpes simplex

ii) palliative in herpes zoster (does not eradicate virus from root ganglia).

Precautions:– may depress liver function and haemopoeisis.

See also:– amantadine, zidovudine.

ADH (ANTIDIURETIC HORMONE; VASOPRESSIN)

Hormone of posterior pituitary. Enhances water reabsorption in distal tubules and collecting ducts. In pharmacological doses constricts resistance vessels via action at vasopressin receptors.

Nonapeptide therefore only effective after injection (or nasal insufflation).

Uses:– replacement therapy in diabetes insipidus.

See also:– desmopressin, felypressin, lypressin, oxytocin.

ADRENALINE

Agonist at α- and β-adrenoceptors (normal transmitter released from adrenal medulla and some neurones in CNS).

Inactivated by:– i) uptake
ii) N-oxidation (MonoAmine Oxidase; MAO)
iii) O-methylation (Catechol-O-Methyl Transferase; COMT).

Uses:– i) to treat allergic emergencies esp. anaphylaxis (dilates airways via β-adrenoceptors & constricts blood vessels via α-adrenoceptors)

ii) as vasoconstrictor **a)** prolongs action of local anaesthetics
b) in bloodless field surgery
c) nasal decongestant
d) slows bleeding from boxing wounds.

Precautions:– once popular use to elevate blood pressure in traumatic shock now considered inadvisable as impairs blood flow to vital organs.

ADRENOCORTICOTROPHIC HORMONE

See **ACTH**.

ALDOSTERONE

Steroid hormone of the adrenal cortex released in response to **ANGIOTENSIN II**; stimulates re-uptake of Na^+ (and hence water) and secretion of K^+ by distal tubules in kidney.

See also:– spironolactone.

ALLOPURINOL

Xanthine-oxidase inhibitor – reduces rate of formation of uric acid from purines.

Uses:– Prophylaxis of gout.

Precautions: i) may cause rashes or gastro-intestinal disorders.
   ii) occasional hypersensitivity reactions occur.
   iii) may interfere with cytotoxic chemotherapy in neoplasic disease.

See also:– colchicine.

ALLOXAN

Selectively destroys B-cells in pancreatic Islets of Langerhans.

Uses:– experimental tool only.

ALPROSTADIL (PROSTAGLANDIN E$_1$)

Agonist at prostaglandin E-type receptors.

Uses:– maintainance of ductus arteriosus patency in neonates before surgery to correct congenital heart defects.

See also:– dinoprost, dinoprostone.

AMANTADINE

Antiviral agent – inhibits entry of some RNA- or DNA-containing virions into host cells.

Also found to be agonist at dopamine receptors.

Uses:– **i)** treatment of viral diseases (A-strain influenza and herpes zoster).
   ii) treatment of Parkinson's disease.

Precautions:– unwanted effects generally extension of drug's action at dopamine receptors.

AMETHOCAINE

As **LIGNOCAINE** but ester and more lipid soluble.

Uses:– as eyedrops to anaesthetise cornea for tonometry, etc.

AMIDOPYRINE
As **ASPIRIN**, but too toxic for use in man.

AMILORIDE
"Potassium-sparing" diuretic. Inhibits Na^+ reabsorption in collecting duct by blocking Na^+ channels. Hence Na^+/K^+ exchange inhibited.

Uses:– to limit K^+ loss during treatment with other diuretics (e.g. **BENDROFLUAZIDE** or **FRUSEMIDE**).

Precautions:– avoid use if plasma K^+ already elevated.

See also:– triamterene.

AMINOBENZOIC ACID
Absorbs solar radiation in the range 290-320 nm.

Uses:– in sun-screen creams and lotions.

p-AMINOBENZOATE
Precursor (with pteridine) of dihydrofolate in bacterial cells. Sulphonamides (e.g. **SULPHAMETHIZOLE**) are structural analogues.

γ-AMINO BUTYRIC ACID
See **GABA**.

AMINOCAPROIC ACID
Inhibits activation of fibrinolysinogen (plasminogen).

Uses:– i) helps staunch bleeding in haemophiliacs after dental extractions
ii) limits fibrinolysis after excessive doses of fibrinolysinogen activators (e.g. **STREPTOKINASE**) in attempts to dissolve fresh thrombi.

Precautions:– may precipitate clot formation in individuals with history of thromboembolic disorders and in pregnancy.

See also:– tranexamic acid.

AMINOGLUTETHIMIDE
Inhibitor of formation of pregnenolone from cholesterol. Hence inhibits production of all steroid hormones. Also inhibits peripheral formation of oestrogen.

Uses:– i) to reduce secretion from autonomously secreting adrenal tumours.
ii) in treatment of post-menopausal breast cancer (**DEXAMETHA-**

SONE also given as replacement for endogenous corticosteroids).

Precautions:– i) signs of adrenal insufficiency predictable untoward effect – hence replacement therapy with glucocorticoid and possibly mineralocorticoid essential
ii) induces hepatic enzymes.

See also:– cyproterone acetate.

AMINO-OXYACETIC ACID

Inhibitor of GABA-transaminase.

Uses:– experimental tool.

AMINOPHYLLINE

As **THEOPHYLLINE**.

Chemically, a complex between **THEOPHYLLINE** and **ETHYLENEDIAMINE**. Much more soluble than **THEOPHYLLINE**.

AMINOPYRINE (USP)

See **AMIDOPYRINE**.

5-AMINOSALICYLATE

As **ASPIRIN**; released by bacterial action in gut lumen from **SULPHASALAZINE**. Not well absorbed hence anti-inflammatory action exerted on gut.

AMIODARONE

Antidysrhythmic drug with complex action (Group 3); prolongs refractory period of cardiac cells (possibly by blocking K^+ channels). Also blocks Na^+ channels.

Unusual pharmacokinetics; may take weeks to reach therapeutic concentrations in plasma and microcrystalline deposits often occur in cornea, skin and other sites – these considerably delay fall of plasma levels once drug is withdrawn. Molecule contains iodine which may be released during metabolism.

Uses:– treatment of supraventricular tachycardias, especially Wolff-Parkinson-White syndrome.

Precautions:– i) released iodine may cause disturbed thyroid function (hypo- or hyper-)
ii) commonly causes photosensitivity of the skin – keep skin covered and use sun-screen ointment (see **AMINOBENZOIC ACID**).

AMITRIPTYLINE

As **IMIPRAMINE**.

AMOXYCILLIN

As **AMPICILLIN** but more lipid soluble therefore absorption after oral administration more reliable.

AMPHETAMINE

See **DEXAMPHETAMINE**.

AMPHONELIC ACID

As **DEXAMPHETAMINE**, but exclusively central action (possibly because selective for dopaminergic neurones).

Uses:– experimental tool.

AMPHOTERICIN

As **NYSTATIN** but lower toxicity allows it to be used by intravenous infusion for the treatment of systemic fungal infections.

Precautions:– i) commonly causes thrombophlebitis at site of infusion.
  ii) dose related, renal toxicity occurs in about 80% of patients; reversible at low doses.
  iii) nausea, vomiting, tinnitus & vision disturbances common.

AMPICILLIN

As **BENZYLPENICILLIN** but wider spectrum. Resistant to gastric acid but sensitive to β-lactamase.

AMYLOBARBITONE

As **DIAZEPAM**, but shorter duration of action (half life ca. 18 h). Chemically a **BARBITURATE**.

ANCROD

Anticoagulant. Enzymic constituent (glycoprotein) of the venom of the Malayan pit viper *(Agkistroden rhodostoma)*. Catalyses the conversion of fibrinogen into an unstable form of fibrin – forms micro-emboli which are dealt with by the reticuloendothelial system (action similar but not identical to thrombin). This depletes fibrinogen levels – hence lower clotting capacity.

Broken down in GI tract therefore must be given by intravenous infusion.

Uses:– treatment of deep-vein thrombosis and prevention of thrombus formation after surgery.

Precautions:– i) haemorrhage extension of desired pharmacological action
ii) formation of thrombo-embolus – extension of desired pharmacological action
iii) anaphylaxis (antigenic as glycoprotein).

ANDROSTENEDIONE

Intermediate in the synthesis of 17-β-**OESTRADIOL** and **TESTOSTERONE** in the ovary and testis.

Uses:– experimental tool only.

ANGIOTENSIN I

Essentially inactive decapeptide formed from inactive **ANGIOTENSINOGEN** (plasma α_2-globulin) by **RENIN**.

Substrate for ACE (Angiotensin Converting Enzyme) – product is **ANGIOTENSIN II**.

Uses:– experimental tool only.

ANGIOTENSIN II

Contracts vascular smooth muscle via angiotensin receptors; most potent pressor agent known. Stimulates **ALDOSTERONE** production and hence Na^+ and water retention.

Nonapeptide formed from **ANGIOTENSIN I** by ACE (Angiotensin Converting Enzyme). Broken down by plasma and tissue aminopeptidases to inactive peptide fragments.

Uses:– experimental tool only.

See also:– angiotensin I, bradykinin, captopril.

ANTHRALIN (USP)

See **DITHRANOL**.

ANTI-DIURETIC HORMONE

See **ADH**.

ANTIPYRINE (USP)

See **PHENAZONE**.

APAMIN

Blocks K^+ channels in cell membranes. Constituent of bee venom.

Uses:– experimental tool.

See also:– cromokalim, TEA.

APAZONE (USP)

See **AZAPROPAZONE**.

APOMORPHINE

Agonist at dopamine receptors especially those of the chemosensitive trigger zone (CTZ).

Chemically related to **MORPHINE**, but devoid of activity at opioid receptors.

Uses:– experimental tool only.

See also:– bromocryptine, levodopa.

APROTININ

Inhibitor of proteolytic enzymes, e.g. **KALLIKREIN, PLASMIN**. Low specificity.

Polypeptide – hence active only after injection.

Uses:– i) treatment of disseminated intravascular coagulation – effectiveness unproven
ii) treatment of acute pancreatitis – effectiveness unproven.

ARACHIDONIC ACID

Precursor of **PROSTAGLANDINS**.

ARGININE VASOPRESSIN

See **ADH**.

ASPIRIN

Inhibits cyclo-oxygenase and therefore reduces formation of prostaglandins. Anti-pyretic action central and may be due to suppression of prostaglandin formation in the brain. Analgesic action may involve central component not due to cyclo-oxygenase inhibition.

Weak acid; non-ionised, lipid-soluble form favoured by acid environment of stomach, but bulk of aspirin absorbed from ileum (alkaline) because of large surface area. Filtered at glomerulus and reabsorption hindered

9

when urine alkaline.

Precautions:— i) mucus production in stomach partly prostaglandin-dependent hence risk of gastric erosion and bleeding. Contraindicated in patients with peptic ulcers

ii) some individuals hypersensitive and develop an anaphylaxis-like reaction (may be fatal), possibly because inhibition of cyclo-oxygenase diverts arachidonic acid pathway towards the leukotrienes

iii) blocks formation of prothrombin by interfering with action of **VITAMIN K**

iv) binds to plasma albumin and therefore displaces more weakly bound acidic drugs

v) high doses stimulate respiration via CNS leading to respiratory alkalosis. Compensatory mechanisms deplete bicarbonate reserves. Higher doses interfere with carbohydrate metabolism and metabolic acidosis develops. Death may result from the acid-base balance disturbance or the respiratory depression that very high doses produce

vi) unlike **PARACETAMOL** and other anti-inflammatory analgesics, may precipitate liver and brain damage in children ill with chicken-pox or influenza (Reye's syndrome).

See also:— benorylate, indomethacin, paracetamol.

ASTEMIZOLE

As **CHLORPHENIRAMINE** but highly polar – hence entry to CNS very slow, therefore minimal sedation.

ATENOLOL

As **PROPRANOLOL** but shows marked selectivity for cardiac β-adrenoceptors (β_1) compared with airways β-adrenoceptors (β_2). Hence smaller risk of bronchospasm.

Poorly lipid soluble – hence entry to CNS very slow; no intrinsic activity; not membrane stabiliser.

ATRACURIUM

As **TUBOCURARINE** but very short duration of action (15-30 min) because eliminated by spontaneous Hofmann degradation and therefore independant of liver or kidney function.

Precautions:— inactivated when mixed with alkaline solutions (e.g. **THIOPENTONE**).

ATROPINE

Competitive antagonist at muscarinic cholinoceptors (actions on CNS manifest as restlessness leading to hallucinations then delirium).

Small doses may cause paradoxical bradycardia in humans by "stimulating" vagal centre in CNS.

Weak base but lipid soluble. (Quaternary derivatives, e.g. atropine methylnitrate & **IPRATROPIUM BROMIDE**, not lipid soluble).

Naturally occurring in solanaceous plants, e.g. deadly nightshade (*Atropa belladonna*).

Uses:— i) anaesthetic pre-medication – dries secretions, prevents vagally induced bradycardia
  ii) to relieve spasms of gut or urinary tract (colic)
  iii) to dilate airways (esp. in bronchitis)
  iv) to treat iridocyclitis
  v) to reduce gastric acid secretion (large doses – rarely used).

Precautions:— may cause retention of urine and precipitate glaucoma in the elderly.

See also:— benzhexol, homatropine, hyoscine, ipratropium, pirenzepine, tropicamide.

AURANOFIN
As **SODIUM AUROTHIOMALATE**.

AUROTHIOGLUCOSE
As **SODIUM AUROTHIOMALATE**.

AZATHIOPRINE
Prodrug of **MERCAPTOPURINE**.

AZLOCILLIN
As **PENICILLIN** but reserved for i.v. treatment of life-threatening infections with *Pseudomonas aeruginosa*.

AZAPROPAZONE
As **ASPIRIN**.

AZIDOTHYMIDINE
See **ZIDOVUDINE**.

AZT
See **ZIDOVUDINE**.

BAL (BRITISH ANTI-LEWISITE)
See **DIMERCAPROL**.

BARBITURATES
Group of general CNS depressants derived from barbituric acid. Now largely displaced by the **BENZODIAZEPINES**, except for a few drugs with specially useful properties, e.g. **PHENOBARBITONE** an anticonvulsant & **THIOPENTONE** for inducing anaesthesia. All barbiturates cause physical dependence and all induce hepatic enzymes.

BATRACHOTOXIN (BaTX)
Toxin from Columbian arrow poison frog *Phyllobates aurotaenia*. Shifts membrane dependence and inactivation characteristics of neuronal Na^+ channels so that they open at resting membrane potential and remain open despite influx of Na^+.

Uses:— experimental tool only.

See also:— aconitine, dicophane, pyrethrin, veratridine.

BECLOMETHASONE
Corticosteroid (see **PREDNISOLONE**) available as polar dipropionate ester – hence poorly absorbed.

Uses:— i) palliative treatment of inflammatory conditions of skin; topical
ii) treatment of moderate to severe asthma; by inhalation.

Precautions:— as **PREDNISOLONE** but risk of adrenal suppression less as poorly absorbed.

BENDROFLUAZIDE
Diuretic. Inhibits Na^+ and Cl^- reabsorption in distal tubule. Hence Na^+/K^+ exchange also inhibited and K^+ loss increases.

Chemically a thiazide. Moderately water soluble therefore accumulates in tubule by filtration. Also secreted by tubule.

Uses:— i) treatment of hypertension
ii) treatment of congestive cardiac failure.

Precautions:— i) causes hypokalaemia and therefore potentiates cardiac glycosides (e.g. **DIGOXIN**)
ii) reducing body water can cause crystallisation of urate in joints of gout sufferers, i.e. precipitates attacks
iii) may elevate blood glucose in diabetics.

See also:— acetazolamide, amiloride, frusemide, spironolactone.

BENORYLATE
Ester of **PARACETAMOL** and **ASPIRIN**.

BENSERAZIDE
Inhibitor of aromatic amino acid decarboxylase (DOPA decarboxylase).

Polar hence does not cross blood-brain barrier, though well enough absorbed from GI tract to produce systemic effect.

Uses:– as adjunct to **LEVODOPA** in the treatment of Parkinson's disease – protects **LEVODOPA** from breakdown in the periphery thus minimising adverse effects (mainly GI) due to accumulation of **DOPAMINE** and minimising the dose of **LEVODOPA** needed.

See also:– carbidopa, selegiline.

BENZHEXOL
As **ATROPINE** but more lipid soluble.

Uses:– treatment of Parkinsonism.

BENZOCAINE
As **LIGNOCAINE**, but an ester and highly lipid soluble.

Uses:– topical anaesthesia especially mucous membranes of mouth. (In some countries permitted for use in lozenges as slimming aid as it renders food tastless and makes eating and swallowing unpleasant!)

BENZODIAZEPINES
Group of general CNS depressants acting partly by a structurally non-specific mechanism and partly through a structurally specific mechanism that involves a receptor associated with the GABA receptor. Binding to the benzodiazepine site modifies the affinity of the GABA receptor and augments Cl^- conductance – hence inhibition of neuronal activity.

Pharmacology essentially identical for all members of the group; usefulness in different conditions depends upon pharmacokinetic differences, i.e. for use as hypnotics, short duration of action (e.g. **TRIAZOLAM**); as sedatives or anxiolytics, intermediate or long duration (e.g. **DIAZEPAM**). High dependence liability. If benefit not obtained within a month it is unlikely that continued administration will be beneficial. The withdrawal syndrome mimics the conditions for which the drugs were originally prescribed – usually acute anxiety and/or insomnia.

All are highly lipid soluble and many are metabolised to active metabolites that have very long half lives (e.g. **DIAZEPAM**).

13

BENZOIC ACID

Fungistatic agent; mechanism of action uncertain.

Uses:– treatment of mild dermatophytoses, usually in ointment in combination with the keratolytic **SALICYLIC ACID**.

See also:– griseofulvin, miconazole, tolnaftate, undecenoates.

BENZOYL CHOLINE

As **ACETYLCHOLINE**. Absorbs UV at 240 nm – forms basis of tests for cholinesterase activity.

See also:– cinchocaine, suxamethonium.

BENZYL BENZOATE

Arachnicide of unknown mechanism of action.

Selective for mites partly because highly polar and therefore not absorbed by host and can therefore be applied in high concentration to the skin.

Uses:– treatment of scabies (infestation with the mite *Sarcoptes scabiei* which lives in the horny layer of the skin).

See also:– monosulfiram.

BENZYLPENICILLIN

Normal form of **PENICILLIN** (see **PENICILLIN** for mechanism of action and summary of all the penicillins).

Highly water soluble.

BEPHENIUM

Agonist at nicotinic cholinoceptors and causes depolarising neuromuscular blockade of skeletal neuro-muscular transmission (flaccid for mammalian, spastic for ascarids).

Quaternary; hence selective for worms as not absorbed from GI tract.

Uses:– treatment of round worm infestations (*Ascaris*).

BETAHISTINE

As **HISTAMINE**; close structural analogue.

BETAMETHASONE

As **BECLOMETHASONE**. Available as polar valerate.

BETAZOLE

As **HISTAMINE**, but selective for histamine H_2 receptors.

BETHANECHOL

As **ACETYLCHOLINE** but selective for muscarinic cholinoceptors and resistant to hydrolysis (spontaneous or by either type of cholinesterase). Shows marked selectivity for M_2 sub-class of muscarinic cholinoceptors. Quaternary.

Uses:– as **CARBACHOL**.

See also:– McN-A-343, pirenzepine.

BETHANIDINE

As **GUANETHIDINE** but does not deplete noradrenaline stores.

BICUCULLINE

Antagonist of **GABA** (competitive) therefore convulsant.

Uses:– as experimental tool only.

BISACODYL

Stimulant purgative. Probably acts by irritating mucosa and thereby stimulating peristalsis by local reflexes.

Intermediate lipid solubility hence partly absorbed. Conjugated in liver and excreted in bile; deconjugated by gut flora.

Uses:– i) relief of constipation (especially when straining at compacted faeces carries risk of causing prolapse of piles)
ii) to empty colon before radiological or endoscopic examination.

Precautions:– i) laxatives should not be used chronically as they empty the bowel thereby delaying the need to defaecate which may cause the user to believe himself constipated again and therefore to take another dose, etc., etc. . . .
ii) should not be used when obstruction suspected.

See also:– danthron, dioctyl sodium succinate, magnesium sulphate, methyl cellulose.

BLEOMYCIN

Generic name for a closely related group of agents obtained from *Streptococcus verticillus*. Chelates Fe^{2+} and this complex then reacts with O_2 releasing superoxide or free radicals which cause fragmentation of DNA and prevent DNA repair. Hence prevents G_2 phase and mitosis. Causes little if any myelosuppression.

Highly water soluble – hence excreted by filtration at glomerulus; must be injected.

Uses:– treatment of squamous cell carcinomas, lymphomas and testicular cancer.

Precautions:– commonly causes pulmonary fibrosis if total dose exceeds 300 mg. May cause mucocutaneous lesions and/or fever.

BOTULINUS TOXIN (BTX)

Exotoxin produced by *Clostridium botulinum*. Binds irreversibly to terminal membrane of cholinergic nerves and prevents release of **ACETYL-CHOLINE** in response to depolarisation. Hence paralysis and death by asphyxia. Also causes agglutination of erythrocytes.

Active by mouth and can cause a kind of food-poisoning known as botulism (Latin *botulus* = sausage). In the West commonest cause is contamination of imperfectly sterilised home bottled or leaky cans of meat or fish.

At least six subtypes of the toxin, for many of which anti-toxins are available.

Uses:–ii) potential military poison – most potent known toxin
    ii) experimental tool.

BRADYKININ

Relaxes vascular smooth muscle, increases capillary permeability, contracts intestinal smooth muscle, augments transmitter release and stimulates sensory nerve endings via B_1 and B_2 receptors.

Nonapeptide formed from kininogen (α_2-globulins) by proteolytic enzyme (**KALLIKREIN**). Substrate for plasma carboxypeptidase and ACE (Angiotensin Converting Enzyme).

Uses:– experimental tool only.

BRETYLIUM

As **GUANETHIDINE** but does not deplete noradrenaline stores.

BROMHEXINE

Causes slow fragmentation of mucopolysaccharide fibres of mucus – hence reduces viscosity of mucus.

Well absorbed.

Uses:– intended to help respiration in compromised patients by facilitating expectoration; unsubstantiated.

BROMOCRYPTINE

Agonist at dopamine receptors. Derivative of ergot.

Highly lipid soluble – hence crosses blood-brain barrier – but metabolised rapidly by liver ("first-pass" effect).

Uses:– i) prevention or suppression of lactation
ii) treatment of hypogonadism or galactorrhoea associated with hyper-prolactinaemia
iii) treatment of Parkinsonism
iv) treatment of acromegaly (in normal subjects stimulation of pituitary dopamine receptors increases growth hormone output but in some acromegalics there is a paradoxical decrease).

Precautions:– may precipitate vasospasm in susceptible individuals.

See also:– apomorphine, ergotamine, levodopa, LSD.

BROMPHENIRAMINE

As **CHLORPHENIRAMINE**, but less potent as sedative. Identical structure, except chlorine replaced by bromine.

BUNGAROTOXINS

A group of polypeptide toxins contained in the venom of an elapid snake (i.e. related to the cobras), the Taiwan banded krait (*Bungarus multicinctus*). There are two major components viz.

i) α-bungarotoxin – non-competitive antagonist at (i.e. binds irreversibly to) nicotinic cholinoceptors of neuromuscular junction
ii) β-bungarotoxin – binds irreversibly to cholinergic nerve terminal membranes and inhibits **ACETYLCHOLINE** release (cf. **BOTULINUS TOXIN**).

Uses:– experimental tools only.

BUPIVACAINE

As **LIGNOCAINE** but slow onset (30 min) and long duration (8 h) of action.

Uses:– long duration makes bupivacaine especially suitable for nerve block, prolonged epidural block (e.g. during childbirth) and spinal anaesthesia.

BUPRENORPHINE

Partial agonist at opioid μ-receptors – hence analgesic but also respiratory depressant and sedative without euphoriant or dysphoriant properties; emetic. Precipitates abstinance syndrome in addicts. Not antagonised by **NALOXONE**. Low dependence liability.

Uses:– as **MORPHINE**.

BUSULPHAN

Alkylates -SH bonds (cf. **CYCLOPHOSPHAMIDE**). Produces minimal platelet depression but some depression of marrow likely.

A dimethanesulphonate derivative, i.e. not a nitrogen mustard; does not ionise and moderate lipid solubility – hence adequately absorbed from the GI tract.

Uses:– treatment of choice for chronic myeloid leukaemia.

Precautions:– i) causes fibrosing alveolitis ("busulphan lung")
ii) may produce irreversible aplasia of bone marrow if excessive myelosuppression is maintained.
iii) may cause skin pigmentation

BUTOBARBITONE

As **DIAZEPAM**, but half life ca. 36 h. Chemically a **BARBITURATE**; highly lipid soluble.

Uses:– obsolete.

C

CAFFEINE

Inhibitor of cAMP phosphodiesterase – hence allows build up of cAMP and augments responses to drugs that stimulate adenylate cyclase. This results in CNS and cardiac stimulation, relaxation of airways smooth muscle and a small diuresis.

A methylxanthine. Highly lipid soluble. Naturally occuring in coffee, tea, cola nuts.

Uses:– i) recreational drug
ii) often included with analgesic in OTC headache remedies; value unproven.

Precautions:– overdose produces insomnia, headache, tachycardia and GI disturbance.

See also:– theobromine, theophylline.

CALCITONIN

The hypocalcaemic hormone produced by parathyroid glands. 32 residue polypeptide.

Uses:– i) treatment of hypercalcaemia associated with malignant disease

ii) to relieve pain and neurological symptoms of Paget's disease of bone.

Precautions:– i) risk of hypersensitivity reaction – test injection advisable

ii) after prolonged use antibodies may be produced that neutralise the hormone.

See also:– salcatonin.

CAPTOPRIL

Analogue of the C-terminal of **ANGIOTENSIN I** but with a sulphydryl group stategically placed to bind irreversibly to the Zn^{2+} atom in the active centre of ACE (Angiotensin Converting Enzyme). Hence inhibits the conversion of inactive **ANGIOTENSIN I** to active **ANGIOTENSIN II** and thus lowers blood pressure.

Uses:– i) treatment of mild to moderate hypertension
  ii) treatment of congestive cardiac failure.

Precautions:– i) may cause precipitous falls in blood pressure in patients with high plasma aldosterone levels (e.g. impaired kidney function, low sodium diets, those taking diuretics or undergoing dialysis)
  ii) higher doses may result in rashes, loss of sense of taste, proteinuria, agranulocytosis, neutropaenia
  iii) some patients develop intractable coughing fits which often terminate in vomiting.

CARBACHOL

As **ACETYLCHOLINE** but resistant to hydrolysis (spontaneous or by either type of cholinesterase).

Quaternary.

Uses:– i) to stimulate contraction of bladder in urinary retention (post-operative or associated with neurological impairment)
  ii) to relieve glaucoma
  iii) to stimulate gut motility in post-operative atony or paralytic ileus.

See also:– bethanechol, DMPP, furtrethonium, methacholine, pilocarpine, TMA.

CARBAMAZEPINE

Anticonvulsant with uncertain mechanism of action – possibly similar to **PHENYTOIN**.

Chemically related to tricyclic antidepressants. Lipid soluble; half life (including active metabolites) moderately long (at least 24 h). Induces hepatic mixed function oxidase system and after chronic treatment, half life may be halved.

Uses:– **i)** treatment of epilepsy, especially partial seizures
  ii) treatment of trigeminal neuralgia (not due to a classical analgesic action).

Precautions:– adverse effects largely extension of desired pharmacology, i.e. blurring of vision, dizziness, drowsiness and ataxia.

CARBARYL
As **PHYSOSTIGMINE**.

Chemically a carbamate, i.e. substituted carbamic acid and therefore highly polar and not absorbed through skin.

Uses:– insecticide in the treatment of pediculosis (infestation with the head or body louse – *Pediculus humanus*) or the crab louse (*Phthirus pubis*).

CARBIDOPA
As **BENSERAZIDE**.

CARBIMAZOLE
Inhibits condensation of mono- and di-iodotyrosine in the thyroid. Also inhibits iodination of tyrosine residues. Hence thyroid hormone production inhibited.

Chemically a thioamide. Lipid soluble and metabolised to active metabolite **METHIMAZOLE**, which is more water soluble (half life of active metabolites ca. 12 h).

Uses:– treatment of hyperthyroidism (diffuse toxic goitre) or preceding surgery for removal of autonomously functioning nodules.

Precautions:– may cause agranulocytosis – ca. 1 in 500 cases. Reversible if treatment stopped.

See also:– potassium perchlorate, propranolol, radioactive iodine.

CARBINOXAMINE
As **CHLORPHENIRAMINE**.

CARBOCISTEINE
Breaks disulphide bonds in mucus, thereby lowering its viscocity.

Uses:– as an aerosol, intended to help respiration in compromised patients by facilitating expectoration; unsubstantiated.

CATECHOL
Inhibitor of COMT.
Uses:– experimental tool only.

CEFUROXIME
As **CEPHRADINE** but less susceptible to β-lactamase and more useful in life-threatening Gram-negative septicaemias.

CEPHALOMYCINS
As **CEPHALOSPORINS.**

CEPHALOSPORINS
Group of antibiotics with close structural resemblance to the **PENICIL-LINS** and similar mechanism of action, e.g. **CEPHRADINE.**

CEPHRADINE
As **AMOXYCILLIN**, but resistant to β-lactamase. Chemically a cephalosporin. Actively secreted by tubules – hence half life less than 1 h.
Precautions:– at least 10% of **PENICILLIN**-hypersensitive patients are hypersensitive to cephalosporins.

CHLORAL HYDRATE
CNS depressant (as **ETHANOL**) – hence sedative and hypnotic.

Water miscible liquid – molecule small enough to allow passage through water-filled pores in cell membranes. Metabolised in liver to active metabolite, **TRICHLOROETHANOL.**
Uses:– i) therapeutically as hypnotic or sedative, especially in children
   ii) nefariously as the original "Micky Finn" knock-out drops.
Precautions:– i) commonly causes gastric irritation – risk reduced if well diluted and if taken only on full stomach. (More palatable complexes that cause less gastric irritation are **DICHLORALPHENAZONE** and **TRICLOFOS SODIUM.**)
   ii) dependence liability similar to **ETHANOL.**

CHLORAMBUCIL
As **CYCLOPHOSPHAMIDE** but slower action.
Uses:– treatment of chronic lymphatic leukaemia.

CHLORAMPHENICOL

Broad spectrum antibiotic – binds to 50S subunit and blocks peptidyl transferase activity.

Lipid soluble.

Uses:– Owing to toxicity reserved for serious life-threatening infections, e.g. *H. influenzae* meningitis and typhoid. Topical use against infections of the eye unlikely to cause serious toxicity.

Precautions:– i) most patients show a dose-related reversible bone marrow depression but approximately 1 in 40,000 develops irreversible and total marrow aplasia – fatal
ii) in neonates impaired handling of glucuronide conjugates may cause "grey baby" syndrome.

CHLORCYCLIZINE

As **CHLORPHENIRAMINE**.

CHLORDIAZEPOXIDE

As **DIAZEPAM**, but shorter duration of action (half life ca. 18 h).

CHLORMETHIAZOLE

CNS depressant (cf. **ETHANOL**). Also inhibits aldehyde dehydrogenase.

Weak base, but with very low pKa (ca. 3). Half-life ca. 4 h.

Uses:– i) sedative and hypnotic
ii) acute phase of withdrawal alcoholics ("detoxification")
iii) to terminate status epilepticus (i.v. injection).

Precautions:– i) may cause thrombophlebitis at site of injection
ii) short half-life may allow status epilepticus to become re-established
iii) risk of respiratory depression
iv) high dependence liability.

CHLOROFORM

Volatile anaesthetic (CNS depressant). Sensitises myocardium to catecholamines (e.g. **NORADRENALINE, ADRENALINE**) – hence risk of sudden cardiac arrest. Also can cause liver necrosis.

Volatile liquid – trichloromethane. Relatively low water solubility therefore induction rapid.

Uses:– obsolete.

CHLOROQUINE

Flat ring of structure intercalates between layers of base pairs in DNA and inhibits transcription (largely by impairing DNA polymerase function). Concentrated in all nucleated cells but selective for malaria cells as these concentrate chloroquine much more than host's cells. Chloroquine also inhibits phospholipase A_2 (higher doses than are antimalarial) – hence anti-inflammatory.

Chemically a 4-aminoquinoline.

Uses:– **i)** prophylactic against malaria

ii) clinical cure of malaria (as *Plasmodium falciparum* has no exoerythrocytic hypnozoites, effects a radical cure of infection with this form)

iii) clearing the blood of *P.vivax*, *P.malariae*, or *P.ovale* prior to attempts at radical cure with **PRIMAQUINE** when the patient is clinically well

iv) treatment of liver abscesses due to *Entamoeba histolytica* – selectivity enhanced as liver cells concentrate chloroquine more than most host cells hence amoeba concentrate chloroquine further by engulfing liver cells

v) as an anti-inflammatory.

Precautions:– retinopathy and rash only likely at high (anti-inflammatory) doses.

See also:– primaquine, quinidine, quinine.

8-CHLOROTHEOPHYLLINE

Chlorinated **METHYLXANTHINE** used to make a more soluble complex with **DIPHENHYDRAMINE**, known as **DIMENHYDRINATE**.

CHLORPHENIRAMINE

Competitive antagonist at histamine H_1 receptors. Also antagonist at muscarinic cholinoceptors and sedative, although chlorpheniramine less potent sedative than other histamine antagonists in most subjects, possibly because more polar.

Moderate lipid solubility – well absorbed and enters CNS.

Uses:– **i)** relief of allergies of upper respiratory tract, eyes and skin

ii) as adjunct to **ADRENALINE** in treatment of anaphylactic shock.

Note:– many of the "anti-histamines" have found use as sedatives, antimotion sickness remedies, nasal decongestants due to their actions at receptors other than histamine receptors (mainly muscarinic cholinoceptors).

Precautions:– **i)** most histamine H_1 receptor antagonists are sedative and therefore interfere with patients' ability to operate complex machinery, including cars; also additive with other sedatives

ii) adverse effects are largely predictable on the basis of the drugs known potency at other receptor types.

See also:– astemizole, chlorpromazine, cimetidine, phenoxybenzamine, terfenadine.

CHLORPROMAZINE

Competitive antagonist at dopamine receptors.

Chemically, a phenothiazine.

Also antagonist at α-adrenoceptors, muscarinic cholinoceptors, histamine H_1 receptors, 5-HT receptors. Inhibits neuronal uptake of **NORADREN-ALINE**. (All these actions detectable at similar concentrations, i.e. low selectivity.)

Lipid soluble.

Uses:– i) neuroleptic esp. in schizophrenia
    ii) useful in the control of nausea and vomiting associated with middle-ear disease, uraemia or chemo/radio-therapy. Also in severe cases of sickness in pregnancy
    iii) persistent hiccups
    iv) termination of "bad trips" following LSD abuse.

Precautions:– most unwanted actions result from extension of normal pharmacology:–
    i) extra-pyramidal symptoms, gynaecomastia and galactorrhoea, hypothermia – via dopamine receptors
    ii) dry mouth, blurred vision, etc. – via cholinoceptors
    iii) hypotension – via α-adrenoceptors.

Prolonged use leads to tardive dyskinesias which may become irreversible. Prolonged use may also lead to abnormal skin pigmentation and photosensitivity.

See also:– flupenthixol, haloperidol, pimozide.

CHLORPROPAMIDE

As **TOLBUTAMIDE** but longer half-life (ca. 36 h).

Precautions:– i) may cause aplastic anaemia (causal link not firmly established)
    ii) may cause an autoimmune haemolytic anaemia.

CHLORTETRACYCLINE

As **TETRACYCLINE** but highly toxic and low lipid solubility.

Uses:– suitable for application to skin and eye as poorly absorbed, hence selectivity enhanced. Useful for treating impetigo. Effective against trachoma.

CHLORTHALIDONE

As **BENDROFLUAZIDE** but longer half life allows dosing on alternate days. Structure related to the thiazides.

CHOLINE THEOPHYLLINATE

As **THEOPHYLLINE** but more soluble salt.

CHORIONIC GONADOTROPHIN

See **HCG**.

CIMETIDINE

Antagonist at H_2 histamine receptors; competitive. Also competes with **TESTOSTERONE** for androgen receptors and can elevate prolactin levels. Sedative.

Highly lipid soluble. Inhibits hepatic MFO system via action on cytochrome P_{450}. Half-life ca. 4 h.

Uses:– i) treatment of peptic ulcer
  ii) treatment of oesophageal reflux
  iii) treatment of Zollinger-Ellison syndrome.

Precautions:– i) risk of impairment of complex motor tasks because of sedative properties
  ii) often causes diarrhoea
  iii) sexual dysfunction (impotence) and gynaecomastia due to interference with **TESTOSTERONE** function and raised **PROLACTIN** levels.

See also:– ranitidine.

CINCHOCAINE

As **AMETHOCAINE**. Also substrate for cholinesterase.

Uses:– forms basis of the **DIBUCAINE** test for atypical cholinesterase (competes with benzoyl choline for enzyme; atypical enzyme is inhibited much less than the normal enzyme). **Note:–** **DIBUCAINE** is the USP name for **CINCHOCAINE**.

See also:– benzoylcholine, suxamethonium.

CINANSERIN

As **CYPROHEPTADINE**, but more selective for 5-HT receptors.

Uses:– experimental tool.

See also:– ketanserin, methysergide.

CINNARIZINE

As **CHLORPHENIRAMINE**, but less selective – antagonist at dopamine receptors and Ca^{2+} channel blocker.

Uses:– i) treatment of motion sickness and nausea and vomiting due to vestibular disease
ii) vasodilator in peripheral vascular disorders – value unproven.

CISPLATIN

As **CYCLOPHOSPHAMIDE** but not a nitrogen mustard. (Cisplatin has two functional chlorides that dissociate and alow the molecule to cross-link the two strands of DNA.)

Uses:– chemotherapy of a wide range of solid tumours.

Precautions:– i) kidney damage likely – minimised by giving plenty of water to drink; monitor creatinine clearance
ii) notorious emetic – hence need, e.g. **METOCLOPRAMIDE**.

CLINDAMYCIN

As **CHLORAMPHENICOL** but does not cause aplastic anaemia. Also concentrates in urine, bile and deposited in bone. Active against *Bacteroides fragilis*, as well as many penicillin-resistant staphylococci.

Uses:– bone and joint staphylococcal infections.

Precautions:– risk of potentially fatal pseudomembranous colitis due to toxin produced by the clindamycin resistant organism, *Clostridium difficile*.

CLOBETASONE BUTYRATE

As **HYDROCORTISONE** but more potent.

CLOMIPHENE

Partial agonist at oestrogen receptors.

Lipid soluble and posesses long half-life.

Uses:– i) induction of ovulation in patients with intact but malfunctioning hypothalamus-pituitary-ovarian axis (e.g. amenorrhoea after oral contraceptives)
ii) in conjunction with HCG to produce multiple ovulation to allow harvesting for in vitro fertilisation.

See also:– cyproterone, tamoxifen.

CLONAZEPAM

As **DIAZEPAM**.

CLONIDINE

Agonist at α-adrenoceptors – highly selective for α_2-adrenoceptors (usually pre-junctional).

Also antagonist at muscarinic cholinoceptors and causes sedation.

Highly lipid soluble (absorbable through skin).

Uses:– treatment of moderate hypertension (action on central neurones involved in control of BP).

Precautions:– sudden withdrawal can precipitate "rebound" hypertensive crisis.

See also:– methyldopa, prazosin, yohimbine.

COCAINE

Blocks Na^+ channels – hence local anaesthetic. Also inhibits $Uptake_1$ into noradrenergic neurones.

Ester and weak base but highly lipid soluble.

Extracted from leaves of South American shrubs *Erythroxylon coca* and *E. truxillense*.

Uses:– i) local anaesthetic (this was the original local anaesthetic). Now obsolete except for topical use in the eye, but only when concommittant vasoconstriction desired
ii) "recreational drug". Effects much as **DEXAMPHETAMINE**. Favoured route of administration is nasal insufflation (classically through a rolled up high denomination bank note). Free base known as **CRACK**
iii) experimental tool for inhibiting noradrenaline disposition into neurones.

Precautions:– i) excessive ocular use can cause corneal ulceration associated with vasoconstriction
ii) high dependence liability, especially if injected i.v. or smoked as free base (**CRACK**).

CODEINE

As **MORPHINE** but probably only partial agonist at μ-receptors, hence maximal analgesic effect less. Also less potent and longer duration of action; has some of the excitant properties of **PETHIDINE**.

COLCHICINE

Disrupts microtubules.

Rapidly absorbed but concentrated in bile and intestinal secretions.

Extracted from the autumn crocus or meadow saffron (*Colchicum autumnale*).

Uses:– Relieves inflammation in gouty arthritis (ineffective in other types of arthritis) – dramatic effect in acute attacks; some prophylactic action (but see below).

Precautions:– toxicity associated with damage to rapidly dividing cells esp. intestinal epithelium (i.v. injection minimises GI toxicity). Chronic use may cause agranulocytosis, aplastic anaemia, myopathy, alopecia, azospermia.

See also:– allopurinol, phenylbutazone.

COLISTIN

Binds to cell membranes and causes damage and cell death. Some selectivity for Gram-negative bacilli. Also antagonist at nicotinic cholinoceptors of skeletal muscle.

A polypeptide antibiotic. Highly water soluble – hence not absorbed from the GI tract.

Uses:– i) treatment of skin infections
ii) treatment of life-threatening infections with *Pseudomonas*.

Precautions:– i) contraindicated in myaesthenia gravis
ii) additive effect with antagonists at nicotinic cholinoceptors may cause excessive paralysis.

CO-PROXAMOL

Compounded analgesic containing **DEXTROPROPOXYPHENE** and **PARACETAMOL** (1:10).

CORTICOSTERONE

Steroid hormone produced by the adrenal cortex.

CORTICOTROPHIN

See **ACTH**.

CORTISOL (USP)

See **HYDROCORTISONE**.

CO-TRIMOXAZOLE

Compounded anti-bacterial preparation comprising **SULPHAMETHA-ZOLE** and **TRIMETHOPRIM** (5:1).

Uses:– i) invasive *Salmonella* infections
ii) *Haemophylus influenzae* infections of joints and bones
iii) resistant infections of the urinary tract

iv) replacement for penicillin in treating certain infections (e.g. gonorrhoea) in penicillin allergic patients.

Precautions:– see constituent drugs.

CRACK
See **COCAINE** (street name for free base form).

CROMOGLYCATE
See **SODIUM CROMOGLYCATE**.

CROMOKALIM
K^+ channel opener. Hyperpolarises vascular smooth muscle – hence smaller contractile responses to spasmogenic influences.

Uses:– under investigation as bronchodilator and hypotensive agent.

See also:– nicorandil, pinacidil.

CROMYLYN SODIUM (USP)
See **SODIUM CROMOGLYCATE**.

CYCLIZINE
As **CHLORPHENIRAMINE** but less selective (higher relative potency at muscarinic cholinoceptors) and potent local anaesthetic.

Chemically a piperazine. Lipid soluble.

Uses:– as **CHLORPHENIRAMINE** but more useful as an anti-emetic.

CYCLOHEXIMIDE
Interferes with cell replication by preventing translocation.

Uses:– experimental tool for inhibiting protein synthesis.

See also:– actinomycin D, bleomycin, doxorubicin.

CYCLOPHOSPHAMIDE
Causes cross-linking of strands of DNA thereby inhibiting transcription – rapidly multiplying cells more susceptible than normal cells.

Moderate lipid solubility; hence active after oral administration. Prodrug which yields alkylating (nitrogen mustard) derivative after metabolism in liver (MFO system).

Uses:– treatment of lymphocytic leukaemia, lymphomas and solid tumours.

Precautions:– i) acrolein is a metabolite and this accumulates in the urine

and can cause haemmorhagic cystitis – minimised if patient given plenty of water to drink. If high doses unavoidable this unwanted effect can be further limited by administration of the neutralising agent **MESNA**
ii) a metabolite denatures cytochrome P_{450} which impaires metabolism of cyclophosphamide itself as well as other drugs.

CYCLOPROPANE

As **HALOTHANE** but gaseous.

Forms explosive mixture with air or oxygen.

CYCLOSERINE

Structural analogue of D-alanine; hence inhibits bacterial cell wall synthesis.

Low molcular weight allows this polar molecule to penetrate water-filled pores in cell membranes – hence well absorbed and equilibrates across tubule.

Uses:– reserved for use in tuberculosis resistant to first-line drugs.

CYPROHEPTADINE

As **CHLORPHENIRAMINE**, but also potent antagonist at 5-HT receptors.

CYPROTERONE

Antagonist at androgen receptors. Also progestogenic.

Lipid soluble.

Uses:–ᅠi) treatment of severe hirsutism due to excessive secretion of androgens by adrenals in women
ii) in combination with an oestrogen for treatment of severe acne in women
iii) attenuation of sexual drive in sexual offenders
iv) second line therapy for prostatic cancer that has metastasised.

Precautions:–ᅠi) adverse effects largely extension of desired pharmacology – development of female hair pattern, gynaecomastia, fat deposition on hips, arrests bone growth and testicular development in immature individuals
ii) predisposes to thrombo-embolism in susceptible individuals.

CYTARABINE

Analogue of pyrimidines that competes with cytidine for base pairing and thereby inhibits DNA synthesis.

Highly polar – hence only effective after injection (usually infusion).

Uses:– palliation of malignant neoplasms – especially acute myeloblastic leukaemia.

Precautions:– causes marked suppression of bone marrow.

DANAZOL

Inhibitor of gonadotrophin release (either selective agonist for pituitary steroid receptors compared with peripheral steroid receptors or agonist with low intrinsic efficacy on peripheral receptors). Possesses some androgenic agonist activity.

Derivative of **ETHISTERONE**, i.e. steroid – highly lipid soluble.

Uses:– treatment of endometriosis, menorrhagia and cystic breast lesions in women and gynaecomastia in men.

Precautions:– adverse effects largely due to androgenic properties eg hair growth, acne and deepening of the voice.

DANTHRON

Irritant purgative. Synthetic – an anthroquinone.

Moderate lipid solubility (may appear in the milk of lactating women). Excretion in urine may colour urine red.

Uses:– i) evacuation of bowel before surgery, endoscopy or radiological examination
ii) treatment of acute constipation.

Precautions:– i) irritation of colon may cause intestinal cramps
ii) may cause intestinal damage if obstruction present
iii) prolonged use may lead to colonic paralysis and loss of potassium.

DANTROLENE

Inhibits release of Ca^{2+} from sarcoplasmic reticulum of skeletal muscle.

Lipid soluble.

Uses:– i) treatment of malignant hyperpyrexia (genetic condition – potentially fatal attacks triggered by, e.g. **SUXAMETHONIUM** in which massive Ca^{2+} release in skeletal muscles causes massive oxidation of ATP and hence heat production)
ii) muscle spasms.

Precautions:– CNS depressant hence risk of sedation, etc. – avoid operation of complex machinery, e.g. motor vehicles.

DAPSONE

Structural analogue of aminobenzoate – hence inhibits dihydrofolate synthetase (cf. **SULPHAMETHIZOLE**). Exhibits selectivity for *Mycoplasma leprae*.

A sulphone. Moderate lipid solubility. Some enteroheparic cycling.

Uses:– i) treatment of leprosy

ii) in combination with inhibitors of dihydrofolate reductase (e.g. **TRIMETHOPRIM**) in treatment of malaria, especially **CHLORO-QUINE**-resistant strains.

D.C.I. (DICHLOROISOPRENALINE)

Partial agonist at β-adrenoceptors – historically the "lead compound" preceding **PROPRANOLOL**.

Uses:– experimental tool.

See also:– acebutalol, pindolol, practolol.

D.D.T.

See **DICOPHANE**.

DEANOL

Precursor of choline; claimed to elevate brain acetylcholine levels and thereby elevating mood and increasing intelligence.

Less polar than choline (tertiary rather than quaternary) but transported by same carriers as choline.

Uses:– experimental tool.

DEBRISOQUINE

As **GUANETHIDINE** but does not deplete noradrenaline stores.

DECAMETHONIUM

Agonist at nicotinic cholinoceptors of skeletal muscle end-plate which therefore causes depolarising blockade of neuromuscular transmission.

A bis-quaternary alkyl ammonium compound – hence not a substrate for cholinesterases and highly water soluble.

Uses:– experimental tool only.

DEHYDROEPIANDROSTERONE

Intermediate in the normal synthesis of **ANDROSTENEDIONE** (and hence **TESTOSTERONE** and **OESTRADIOL**).

DEOXYCORTONE PIVALATE

As **FLUDROCORTISONE** but very low solubility – hence suitable for depot injections.

DEPRENYL (USP)

See **SELEGILINE**.

DESFERRIOXAMINE

Chelating agent with selectivity for iron.

Uses:– i) treatment of poisoning with iron salts
ii) removal of excess Fe^{2+} following multiple transfusion treatment of anaemias.

DESIPRAMINE

Active desmethylated metabolite of **IMIPRAMINE**.

DESMOPRESSIN

Analogue of **ADH** but highly selective for **ADH** receptors in the kidney – hence stimulates water reabsorption with minimal vasoconstriction.

Synthetic peptide and more resistant to enzymic degradation than natural **ADH**.

Uses:– treatment of diabetes insipidus.

See also:– felypressin, oxytocin.

DEXAMETHASONE

As **PREDNISOLONE** but very resistant to metabolism and extensively bound – hence half-life in excess of 2 days.

DEXAMPHETAMINE

As **EPHEDRINE** but very lipid soluble hence predominant CNS actions. Only fair substrate for $Uptake_1$ – gains access to noradrenergic, adrenergic and dopaminergic neurones mainly by rapid diffusion.

CNS effects – activation, increased attention span, resistance to fatigue, anorexia, insomnia, stereotypy and paranoia.

Uses:– i) narcolepsy
ii) increases attention span in "hyperactive" children
iii) once popular as anorectic (short-term loss of a few kg but weight soon replaced).

Precautions:– high abuse liability.

See also:– cocaine, ephedrine, tyramine.

DEXTROMETHORPHAN

As **MORPHINE** but almost devoid of analgesic, addictive and euphoriant activity, i.e. highly selective cough suppressant.

(+)-isomer of O-methylated derivation of **LEVORPHANOL**.

Uses:– suppression of dry, unproductive cough that is disturbing sleep or causing excessive irritation of the respiratory tract.

DEXTROMORAMIDE

As **MORPHINE** but less sedating and shorter half-life.

DEXTROPROPOXYPHENE

As **MORPHINE** but much lower maximal analgesic effect and lower potency but longer half-life.

See also:– co-proxamol.

DEXTRORPHAN

(+)-isomer of **LEVORPHANOL**. Devoid of analgesic activity.

DIAMORPHINE

(Also more popularly known as **HEROIN**). As **MORPHINE** but more euphoriant and higher addiction liability but causes less stimulation of vomiting centre and less constipation.

Subject to considerable "first pass" metabolism in liver if given orally.

MORPHINE is an active metabolite of diamorphine (by de-acetylation).

DIAZEPAM

Anxiolytic-sedative-hypnotic (once confusingly referred to as a "minor tranquilliser"). Combines with an accessory site on chloride channel-linked GABA-receptors and augments affinity for **GABA** and hence increases chloride conductance.

All **BENZODIAZEPINES** have dependence liability – severity of withdrawal syndrome depends upon length of administration (unlikely to be a problem if taken for less than one month), dose and half-life (the shorter the half-life the more severe the syndrome). The abstinence syndrome commonly mimics the original presenting symptoms, i.e. acute anxiety syndrome.

Chemically a **BENZODIAZEPINE**. Highly lipid soluble. Half-life of diazepam and its active metabolites (principally **NORDIAZEPAM**) is very long – approximately 5 days. Final excretion products are mainly conjugates.

Uses:– i) treatment of acute anxiety syndrome
  ii) anti-convulsant in status epilepticus (i.v.)

iii) relief of muscle spasm.

Precautions:– i) if anxiety syndrome is not improved after one month it is unlikely to improve on continued diazepam treatment and the risk of dependence increases dramatically
ii) long half-life means that accumulation will occur (steady state will only be reached after about one month, i.e. 6 half-lives, and the drug will persist for a similar time after dosing stops)
iii) stimulates appetite which may result in weight gain (which may have psychological consequences)
iv) effects additive with other CNS depressants, e.g. **ETHANOL**
v) impairs ability to operate complex machinery, e.g. motor vehicles.

See also:– see under **BARBITURATES, BENZODIAZEPINES**.

DIAZOXIDE

Relaxes vascular smooth muscle, possibly by interfering with ionic movements across smooth muscle cell walls. Also causes Na^+ and water retention – hence interferes with the action of thiazide diuretics, e.g. **BENDROFLUAZIDE**. Also diabetogenic.

Chemically closely related to the thiazide diuretics.

Uses:– i) treatment of hypertensive crises
ii) treatment of chronic hypoglycaemia associated with excessive **INSULIN** secretion.

DIBENAMINE

As **PHENOXYBENZAMINE** (a 2-halo-alkylamine).

DIBUCAINE (USP)

See **CINCHOCAINE**.

DICHLORALPHENAZONE

More soluble, less irritant derivative of **CHLORAL HYDRATE**.

DICOPHANE (DDT)

Increases the time that Na^+ channels in nerves stay open during action potential. Also inhibits K^+ movement through K^+ channels. Hence repolarisation delayed and repetitive firing results, leading to paralysis.

Highly permeant through chitin of insect exoskeleton; much less permeant through mammalian skin (unless in organic solvent). Hence selectively toxic to insects, etc. Selectively accumulates in mammalian fat stores. Very resistant to metabolism (and chemical degradation in the environment).

Uses:– Insecticide, though WHO recommends the use of alternatives because of the persistance of dicophane.

Precautions:– Starvation and the subsequent mobilisation of body fat may lead to the appearance of toxic concentrations of dicophane in the blood.

DICYCLOMINE

As **ATROPINE** but less potent. Also possesses direct smooth muscle relaxing properties.

Tertiary amine.

DIENOESTROL

As **STILBOESTROL**.

DIETHYL ETHER

As **HALOTHANE** but no cardiac sensitisation or liver damage on repeated administration.

High solubility in blood therefore long induction time.

Precautions:– i) vapour forms explosive &/or flammable mixture with oxygen
ii) causes marked irritation of airways resulting in copious salivation and mucus production
iii) high risk of vomiting.

(Once bottle opened risk of peroxide formation on storage – increases explosion risk and irritancy.)

DIETHYLCARBAMAZINE

Antifilarial – acts by increasing susceptibility of organisms to macrophages; precise mechanism unknown. Also agonist at nicotinic cholinoceptors (concentrations higher than those achieved therapeutically).

Chemically a piperazine. Well absorbed from GI tract.

Uses:– treatment of filarial infections; generally effective against both microfilariae and adult forms, but less effective against adult forms of *Onchocerca volvulus*.

Precautions:– i) risk of anaphylactic-type reaction in response to release of proteins from phagocytosed worms; minimised by giving small but progressively increasing doses
ii) commonly causes alopecia.

DIETHYLPROPION
As **DEXAMPHETAMINE**.

DIETHYLSTILBESTROL (USP)
See **STILBOESTROL**.

DIFLUNISAL
As **ASPIRIN** (chemically diflunisal is simply a substituted derivative of **SALICYLIC ACID**). Longer duration of action than **ASPIRIN** and less irritation.

DIGOXIN
Inhibitor of Mg^{2+}-dependent Na^+/K^+-ATPase in myocardial cells. Enzyme inhibition leads to a loss of K^+ and an accumulation of Na^+ inside membrane. This latter may facilitate Ca^{2+} entry and thereby augments contraction of myocardial cells. In nodal cells, ionic changes render cells less excitable leading to block of conduction – beneficial in atrial fibrillation. In Purkinje fibres and bundle of His, membrane potential fall renders cells hyperexcitable and ectopic pacemakers may develop which may lead to ventricular dysrhythmias (possibly fatal). Digoxin also sensitises SA node muscarinic cholinoceptors and causes an increased outflow from the vagal centre in the medulla.

Active part of molecule is a lipid soluble steroid nucleus linked to a highly water soluble sugar moeity. Whole molecule not particularly soluble in either water or lipid. Absorption from GI tract incomplete (ca.60%). Highly protein bound – V_d about 5 l/kg. 90% excreted unchanged in the urine – filtration plus some secretion. Long half life (1–2 days) results from large V_d.

Uses:– i) to increase cardiac output in congestive cardiac failure
ii) in atrial fibrillation (reduces the number of atrial action potentials that successfully traverse the AV node).

Precautions:– i) very small therapeutic index – hence adverse effects occur with only small excesses
ii) most adverse effects extension of desired pharmacology (inhibition of ATPase) – primarily dysrhythmia
iii) dysrhythmogenic actions augmented by low extracellular K^+ – hence beware diuretics, e.g. **BENDROFLUAZIDE**
iv) commonly causes malaise, nausea, vomiting and disturbed colour vision.

DIHYDROCODEINE
As **CODEINE**.

5-α-DIHYDROTESTOSTERONE

Active metabolite of **TESTOSTERONE** formed in target tissues.

DIHYDROXYPHENYLALANINE

See **LEVODOPA**.

DILANOXIDE FUROATE

Amoebicide; mechanism of action uncertain, but presumably selective for parasites because well absorbed and excreted in urine of host.

Uses:– to eliminate *Entamoeba histolytica* from intestine and to prevent host becoming a carrier after clinical signs of infection have been abolished.

DIMAPRIT

Agonist at histamine receptors – highly selective for H_2 receptors (ca. 2000-fold).

Uses:– experimental tool only.

DIMENHYDRINATE

Salt formed between **DIPHENHYDRAMINE** and **8-CHLORO-THEOPHYLLINE**.

Longer duration of action than **DIPHENHYDRAMINE**.

Uses:– motion sickness.

DIMERCAPROL

Dithiol-containing chelating agent with affinity for heavy metal ions eg antimony, arsenic, gold, mercury.

Also known as **BAL** – (British Anti-Lewisite).

Polar – hence given by injection (intramuscular in oil).

Uses:– i) treatment of heavy metal poisoning – prolonged treatment may be required as affinity for metals not greatly more than affinity of tissue sulphydryl groups for the metal ions
ii) treatment of Wilson's disease (chelates surplus copper)
iii) antidote to the chemical warfare agent **LEWISITE**.

Precautions:– should not be used to treat poisoning with cadmium, iron or selenium as the chelates formed are more toxic than the metal ions themselves.

See also:– EDTA, lewisite, penicillamine.

DINOPROST (PROSTAGLANDIN PGF$_{2\alpha}$)

Agonist at prostaglandin F-type receptors.

Very labile – hence administered by intravenous infusion.

Uses:– **i)** termination of pregnancy in 2nd trimester
ii) to cause involution of corpus luteum in domestic animals (eg sheep, cattle) and hence to synchronise oestrus.

Precautions:– **i)** risk of uterine rupture if obstruction to birth canal
ii) can precipitate asthma attacks (brochoconstriction).

DINOPROSTONE (PROSTAGLANDIN E$_2$)

Agonist at prostaglandin receptors of the E type.

Uses:– Induction of labour at term and abortion in second trimester.

Precautions:– adverse effects largely extensions of the normal pharmacology of the drug, e.g. nausea, vomiting, diarrhoea, flushing, headache, dizziness.

DIOCTYL SODIUM SUCCINATE

Emollient laxative. Probably acts by lowering surface tension of gut contents.

DIPHENHYDRAMINE

As **CHLORPHENIRAMINE**. Chemically an oxyethylamine.

DIPHENOXYLATE

Agonist at opioid μ-receptors.

Highly water soluble, hence after oral administration exerts main activity locally in gut wall.

Uses:– anti-diarrhoeal agent.

Precautions:– **i)** as **MORPHINE**
ii) as only commercially available preparation (Lomotil) contains **ATROPINE**, adverse effects may result from antagonism at muscarinic cholinoceptors.

DIPYRIDAMOLE

Inhibits phosphodiesterase of platelets, hence allows cAMP concentrations within platelets to rise, thereby reducing platelet adhesiveness.

Uses:– in conjunction with anti-coagulants to limit formation of clots on artificial heart valves.

Precautions:– adverse effects largely extension of desired pharmacology, e.g. hypotension and throbbing headache. (May precipitate angina attacks in sufferers by dilating branches of coronary artery that supply non-compromised parts of the myocardium.)

DISULFIRAM

Inhibitor of aldehyde dehydrogenase.

Lipid soluble.

Uses:– aversion therapy of alcohol addiction.

Precautions:– i) the small amounts of alcohol used in many medicines (POM and OTC) may be sufficient to cause unpleasant effects
ii) impairs function of dopamine β-oxidase (by chelating copper prosthetic group).

See also:– metronidazole, monosulfiram.

DITHRANOL

Irritant anti-psoriatic. Believed to act by depressing mitosis through interaction with DNA.

Moderately water soluble; hence after topical application, concentrations in skin higher than systemic concentrations.

Uses:– treatment of psoriasis.

Precautions:– some patients are hypersensitive and normal skin is more sensitive to irritant effects than affected skin.

D.M.P.P. (1,1-DIMETHYL-4-PHENYLPIPERAZINIUM)

As **NICOTINE**.

Quaternary.

Uses:– experimental tool only.

DOBUTAMINE

As **DOPAMINE** (but not physiological transmitter).

DOMPERIDONE

Antagonist at dopamine receptors.

Modest lipid solubility therefore does not reach high concentrations in CNS (actions mainly via dopamine receptors of CTZ).

Uses:– treatment of nausea and vomiting, especially as a result of chemotherapy with cytotoxic drugs.

Precautions:– adverse effects largely extensions of normal pharmacology, e.g. galactorrhoea.

DOPA (DIHYDROXYPHENYLALANINE)

See **LEVODOPA**.

DOPAMINE

Normal transmitter in some CNS neurones esp. in striatum. Formed by decarboxylation of DOPA (**LEVODOPA**). Agonist at dopamine receptors, β- and α-adrenoceptors (shows some selectivity for cardiac β-adrenoceptors and perhaps increases force at doses that do not increase rate).

Too polar to cross blood-brain barrier.

Uses:– treatment of cardiogenic shock.

Precautions:– i) often causes vomiting (via CTZ)
   ii) exacerbates Raynaud's syndrome
   iii) may cause dangerous tachycardia at higher doses.

See also:– dobutamine, isoprenaline.

DOXAPRAM

Stimulates respiration, possibly by increasing sensitivity of peripheral chemoreceptors.

Uses:– stimulation of respiration in patients with hypercapnic depression of respiration.

Precautions:– overdose causes non-selective stimulation of CNS leading to convulsions.

See also:– nikethamide.

DOXORUBICIN

Cytotoxic agent which inhibits DNA replication (intercalates in the DNA helix and inhibits transcription).

Uses:– treatment of acute myeloid leukaemia, the lymphomas and some solid tumours.

Precautions:– highly toxic to all tissues and irritant, therefore usually given in fast running intravenous drip. High risk of cardiac myopathy. Adverse effects extensions of desirable pharmacology; rapidly dividing cells most susceptible.

DOXYCYCLINE

As **TETRACYCLINE**, but less risk of renal impairment.

DROPERIDOL

As **HALOPERIDOL**.

DYFLOS

Organophosphorus cholinesterase inhibitor. Binds irreversibly to esteratic site of both acetylcholinesterase (AChE) and butyrylcholinesterase (ChE), but higher affinity for butyrylcholinesterase (ca. 250-fold). Displaceable by strongly nucleophyllic agents, e.g. **PRALIDOXIME** for a short time, after which an irreversible conformational change occurs in the enzyme and the binding becomes irreversible.

Developed prior to World War II as a chemical weapon ("nerve gas").

E

ECHOTHIOPATE

See **ECOTHIOPATE**.

ECHOTHIOPHATE (USP)

See **ECOTHIOPATE**.

ECOTHIOPATE

Irreversible inhibitor of cholinesterase. Close stuctural similarity to acetylcholine. Relatively high selectivity for cholinesterase.

Quaternary.

Uses:– as eye-drops to reduce intraocular pressure in glaucoma.

Precautions:– sufficient drug may be absorbed from the conjunctival sac to produce signs and symptoms of systemic poisoning.

EDROPHONIUM

As **NEOSTIGMINE** but very short duration of action. Non-ester – hence combines only with anionic site of acetylcholinesterase.

Uses:– diagnosis of myaesthenia gravis.

EDTA (ETHYLENEDIAMINETETRA-ACETIC ACID)

Chelator of metal ions. Derivative of **ETHYLENEDIAMINE**. (Others are triethylenetetramine HCl, and calcium pentetate). Usually used as the calcium disodium salt (calcium disodium edetate).

Uses:– i) treatment of heavy metal poisoning, especially lead
ii) anticoagulant (*in vitro*)
iii) pharmacological tool.

EGTA (ETHYLENE GLYCOL-bis(β-AMINOETHYL ETHER) N,N,N',N'-TETRA-ACETIC ACID)

As **EDTA**, but highly selective for Ca^{2+}.

Uses:– experimental tool.

EGTAZIC ACID

See **EGTA**.

ENALAPRIL

As **CAPTOPRIL**.

ENFLURANE

As **HALOTHANE**. Less cardiac sensitisation. Liver damage on repeated administration less likely.

EPHEDRINE

Indirect sympathomimetic, i.e. causes release of endogenous **NORADRENALINE**. Hence non-selective.

Substrate for $Uptake_1$. Relatively non-polar. Resistant to COMT, MAO and $Uptake_2$.

Occurs naturally in shrubs of the genus Ephedra, e.g. *E. sinica* (Ma Huang), indigenous to China.

Uses:– i) bronchodilator in asthma (now obsolete; see **SALBUTAMOL**)
    ii) nasal decongestant (systemic or topical)
    iii) occasionally useful in reducing nocturnal bed-wetting in children (by contracting bladder sphincter and decreasing depth of sleep).

Precautions:– i) insomnia
    ii) potentially dangerous cardiac stimulation.

See also:– dexamphetamine, noradrenaline, phenylephrine, phenyl propanolamine, tyramine.

EPOPROSTENOL

See **PROSTACYCLIN**.

EPSOM SALTS

See **MAGNESIUM SULPHATE**.

ERGOMETRINE

Oxytocic agent. One of the **ERGOT ALKALOIDS** (from the fungus

Claviceps purpura), but very low potency at α-adrenoceptors.

Highly lipid soluble.

Uses:– to accelerate 3rd stage of labour and to limit post-partum bleeding.

Precautions:– i) despite low potency at α-adrenoceptors, vasoconstriction and hypertension can occur
ii) nausea and vomiting not uncommon (presumably by action at dopamine receptors of CTZ).

See also:– ergotamine, LSD, oxytocin.

ERGOT ALKALOIDS

Group of alkaloids naturally occurring in the rye fungus, *Claviceps purpura*. Responsible for outbreaks of "ergotism" in the Middle Ages. The active ingredients are derivatives of lysergic acid amide, e.g. **ERGOMETRINE, ERGOTAMINE**. Many synthetic derivatives have been synthesised, including **BROMOCRYPTINE** & **LSD**.

ERGOTAMINE

Partial agonist at α-adrenoceptors (intrinsic activity ca. 30%). Also antagonist at 5-HT receptors, possibly agonist or partial agonist at dopamine receptors in CNS.

One of the ergot alkaloids extracted from the fungus *Claviceps purpura*.

Uses:– useful for terminating headache in migraine (constricts dilated scalp vessels). Does not modify prodromal phase or neurological components.

Precautions:– prolonged usage or overdose causes intense vaso constriction of extremities leading to gangrene.

See also:– bromocryptine, ergometrine, LSD, methysergide.

ERGONOVINE (USP)

See **ERGOMETRINE**.

ERYTHROMYCIN

Antibiotic. Blocks protein synthesis by binding to 50S subunit of ribosome and preventing translocation. Spectrum similar to **BENZYL-PENICILLIN** but also active against penicillinase-producing strains of *Staphylococcus* and against *Campylobacter*, *Legionella* and *Mycoplasma*.

Moderate lipid solubility (absorbed after oral administration, but penetrates CSF poorly). Metabolised and excreted in bile and urine.

Uses:– i) as alternative to **PENICILLIN** in allergic individuals
ii) treatment of Legionnaires' disease

iii) prophylaxis against whooping cough and diphtheria.

Precautions:– prolonged use of the estolate derivative should be avoided as this may cause cholestatic jaundice.

ETHACRYNIC ACID
As **FRUSEMIDE**.

ETHAMBUTOL
Anti-tubercular drug of unknown mechanism of action. Tuberculostatic.

Absorbed after oral administration but most of the dose excreted unchanged in the urine.

Uses:– in combination with **RIFAMPICIN** and **ISONIAZID** in the treatment of tuberculosis ("triple therapy").

Precautions:– i) dose must be reduced in patients with impaired kidney function
ii) blood concentrations at the top of the therapeutic range can cause vision defects – loss of acuity and colour vision; reversible at first, but may become irreversible.

See also:– streptomycin.

ETHANOL
Non-specific CNS depressant. Anaesthetic dose very close to respiratory depressant dose, hence useless as general anaesthetic.

Highly polar molecule (miscible with water in all proportions), but small enough to cross membranes through water filled pores. Hence distributes rapidly through total body water. Metabolised in liver by alcohol dehydrogenase followed by aldehyde dehydrogenase. Alcohol dehydrogenase saturates at very low concentrations so that metabolism is essentially zero order (rate equivalent to elimination of one unit of alcohol per hour).

Uses:– i) "recreational drug"
ii) sterilising agent (most effective at 70%)
iii) sedative (major constituent of gripe waters)
iv) solvent in many medicinal preparations.

Precautions:– i) withdrawal syndrome in addicts (alcoholics) can be severe ("delirium tremens")
ii) prolonged consumption causes liver cirrhosis
iii) small amounts interfere with ability to operate complex machinery (e.g. cars) safely – effects marked at doses much less than those needed to cause drunkeness
iv) sedative effects additive with other CNS depressant drugs, e.g. **DIAZEPAM**.

ETHER
See **DIETHYL ETHER**.

ETHINYLOESTRADIOL

Agonist at oestrogen receptors, i.e. an oestrogen.

Semi-synthetic steroid; 17-ethinyl group renders the molecule relatively resistant to hepatic metabolism, hence no first-pass effect on oral administration.

Uses:– i) oestrogenic component of oral contraceptives
ii) replacement therapy (not normally for prolonged replacement after the menopause, may be effective in small doses to minimise the impact & may prove beneficial in cases of severe osteoporosis) – most effective when given in combination with a progestagen
iii) treatment of menstrual disorders – most effective when given in combination with a progestagen.

Precautions:– i) prolonged administration may predispose to endometrial carcinoma
ii) may exacerbate diabetes, epilepsy, migraine, hypertension
iii) increases levels of hormone binding protein and may therefore interfere with thyroid or adrenal cortex function tests
iv) large doses increase risk of thrombo-embolism.

ETHISTERONE

Progestagen with marked androgenic activity. Semi-synthetic steroid.

Uses:– experimental tool.

ETHOSUXIMIDE

As **PHENYTOIN** but relatively selective for absence seizures.

Metabolism is first order; induces hepatic enzymes and precipitates porphyria.

ETHYL ALCOHOL
See **ETHANOL**.

ETHYLENE DIAMINE
See **EDTA**.

FELYPRESSIN

Synthetic peptide analogue of **VASOPRESSIN** (see **ADH**).

Uses:– as vasoconstrictor in local anaesthetic solutions.

FENCAMFAMIN

As **DEXAMPHETAMINE**.

Uses:– experimental tool only; obsolete as therapeutic agent.

FENFLURAMINE

Stimulant in CNS (cf. **DEXAMPHETAMINE**), but highly selective appetite suppressant action, probably due to selectivity for 5-HT neurones. Anoretic action is not sustained for more than a few weeks. Despite similarity to **DEXAMPHETAMINE**, fenfluramine has marked sedative properties.

Uses:– short term as adjunct to dietary control in treatment of obesity.

Precautions:– additive sedation with non-specific depressants, e.g. **ETHANOL**.

FENOPROFEN

As **ASPIRIN** but less risk of inducing Reye's syndrome.

FENOTEROL

As **SALBUTAMOL** but less selectivity for airways.

FIBRINOLYSIN

See **PLASMIN**.

FLUCLOXACILLIN

As **BENZYLPENICILLIN**, but resistant to both gastric acid and β-lactamase.

Polar – hence absorption after oral administration variable and not complete.

Precautions:– adequate absorption after oral administration should not be relied upon in seriously ill patients.

FLUDROCORTISONE

Synthetic adreno-cortical steroid. Selective mineralocorticoid rather than glucocorticoid (ca. 12-fold).

Uses:– replacement therapy in adrenocortical insufficiency – most effective in combination with glucocorticoid, e.g. **HYDROCORTISONE**.

Precautions:– adverse effects predictable consequences of the drug's pharmacology
  i) retension of sodium and water – hence hypertension
  ii) loss of potassium
  iii) stunting of growth in children
  iv) further suppression of adrenal cortex (via hypophysis)
  v) increased risk of peptic ulceration.

FLUOROURACIL

Inhibitor of nucleic acid synthesis. A purine analogue – produces false nucleotide that prevents normal deoxyribonucleotide production.

Polar, but transported by the same mechanisms that transport normal purines.

Uses:– palliative treatment of malignant neoplasms.

Precautions:– toxicity largely due to extension of desired pharmacology, e.g. damage to fast growing cell types.

FLUPENTHIXOL

As **CHLORPROMAZINE** but higher selectivity for dopamine receptors.

A thioxanthine.

FLURAZEPAM

As **DIAZEPAM**, but half life ca. 72 h.

FLURBIPROFEN

As **ASPIRIN**, but less risk of inducing Reye's syndrome.

FOLINIC ACID

Precursor of tetrahydrofolate in the synthetic pathway of thymidine.

FRUSEMIDE

Inhibits reabsorption of ions in the thick ascending limb of the loop of Henle. Hence Na^+ and Cl^- enter distal tubule at high concentration, so that less water is resorbed. K^+ is therefore lost as well as Na^+ and Cl^-. Massive, brief diuresis follows. Member of group known as "High Ceiling" or "Loop" diuretics.

Well absorbed from gut, but being acidic, binds to plasma proteins. Enters proximal tubule by filtration and secretion. Short duration of action because i) passively removed from tubule ii) compensatory mechanisms activated.

Uses:– to produce rapid water loss.

Precautions:– hypokalaemia.

See also:– amiloride, bendrofluazide, spironolactone.

FSH (FOLLICLE STIMULATING HORMONE)

Pituitary gonadotrophin responsible for initiating and supporting the growth of Graaffian follicles in the ovary (hence ova and **17-β-OES-TRADIOL**).

FUROSEMIDE (USP)

See **FRUSEMIDE**.

FURTRETHONIUM

As **ACETYLCHOLINE** but selective for muscarinic cholinoceptors. Quaternary. Not an ester.

Uses:– as **CARBACHOL**.

G

GABA (γ-AMINO BUTYRIC ACID)

Inhibitory transmitter in CNS – receptor part of or linked to Cl^- channel.

GALLAMINE

As **d-TUBOCURARINE** but does not evoke **HISTAMINE** release and shorter duration of action.

Also antagonist at muscarinic cholinoceptors.

GAMMA AMINO BUTYRIC ACID

See **GABA**.

GASTRIN

Hormone released locally in stomach; involved in the production of gastric acid.

See also:– pentagastrin.

GENTAMICIN

An aminoglycoside antibiotic. Bactericidal. Spectrum – many Gram-negative and some Gram-positive organisms. Also active against *Pseudomonas aeruginosa*. If given with a **PENICILLIN** also kills *Streptococcus faecalis*.

Highly polar. Hardly metabolised.

Precautions:– i) ototoxicity (plasma concentration should be kept between 2 and 10 mg/l)
ii) impairs neuromuscular transmission (cf. **d-TUBOCURARINE**)
iii) elimination half-time (normally ca. 2 h) increased when renal function impaired.

See also:– kanamycin, neomycin, streptomycin.

GLIBENCLAMIDE

As **TOLBUTAMIDE** but longer half-life (ca. 10 h).

GLICAZIDE

As **TOLBUTAMIDE** but shorter half-life (ca. 4 h).

GLIPIZIDE

As **TOLBUTAMIDE** but longer half-life (ca. 12 h).

GLUCAGON

Pancreatic hormone responsible for rise in blood glucose levels. Glucagon is a 29 unit polypeptide.

GLYCERYL TRINITRATE

Smooth muscle relaxant – possibly acts by elevating intracellular concentrations of cyclic-GMP. Vasodilator, with some selectivity for capacitance vessels over resistance vessels – hence reduces pre-load on heart.

Chemically also known as nitroglycerin – explosive, but safe for medicinal use when adsorbed onto mannitol or lactose and compressed into tablets. Hydrolysed during absorption through gastric mucosa – hence inactive if swallowed, but effective if absorbed through buccal mucosa.

Uses:– **i)** to terminate attacks of angina of effort
ii) treatment of heart failure.

Precautions:– adverse effects extensions of desired pharmacology, i.e. throbbing headache, flushing, hypotension, reflex tachycardia.

See also:– isosorbide dinitrate, nifedipine, propranolol, sodium nitroprusside.

GLYCINE

Inhibitory transmitter in CNS, e.g. Renshaw cells of spinal cord.

See also:– strychnine.

GOLD

See **SODIUM AUROTHIOMALATE**.

GOLD SODIUM THIOMALATE

See **SODIUM AUROTHIOMALATE**.

GRISEOFULVIN

Anti-fungal agent (active against the dermatophytes *Trichophyton, Epidermophyton* & *Microsporum*).

Very lipid soluble (absorption accelerated by fatty meals as absorbed in chylomicrons). Potent inducer of hepatic oxidase system. Sequestered in keratinous tissues after oral administration.

Extracted from the mould *Penicillium janezewski*.

Uses:– Tinea of hair, skin & nails.

Precautions:– **i)** must be administered until all infected keratin has been shed otherwise risk of re-infection
ii) may cause photosensitivity
iii) potent enzyme inducer – hence may precipitate attacks in acute intermittant porphyria.

GROWTH HORMONE (SOMATOTROPHIN)

Pituitary hormone responsible for growth to adult size.

Uses:– use in therapy replaced by **SOMATREM**, human sequence growth hormone produced using recombinant gene technology.

GTN

See **GLYCERYLTRINITRATE**.

GUANETHIDINE

Noradrenergic neurone blocking agent. Drug is local anaesthetic that is accumulated by noradrenergic neurones to effective concentrations – hence selectively impairs transmission in noradrenergic neurones.

Uses:– **i)** glaucoma (as eye-drops)
ii) severe, refractory hypertension.

Precautions:– i) postural hypotension, diarrhoea & impaired ejaculation are unavoidable consequences of the drug's pharmacology
ii) prolonged administration at high doses can lead to accumulation in storage vesicles and depletion of noradrenaline stores
iii) requires neuronal noradrenaline uptake pump (competes with other drugs for uptake).

See also:– bethanidine, bretyllium, debrisoquine, reserpine.

H

HALOPERIDOL

As **CHLORPROMAZINE** but more selective for dopamine receptors.
A butyrophenone.

HALOTHANE

Volatile general anaesthetic.

Also impairs transmission at skeletal neuromuscular junctions & sensitises heart to sympathomimetics (possibly by inhibiting uptake).

Precautions:– repeated administration within 6 weeks may cause irreversible liver failure.

See also:– diethyl ether, enflurane, methoxyflurane, nitrous oxide.

HCG (HUMAN CHORIONIC GONADOTROPHIN)

Hormone produced by chorionic membrane which maintains the corpus luteum during the first trimester, i.e. **LH**-like.

Protein.

Uses:– i) stimulation of ovulation in infertile women who produce low levels of pituitary gonadotrophins. Used in conjunction with **FSH**

ii) possibly of value to enhance testosterone production in delayed puberty

iii) in conjunction with **FSH** may increase sperm count in infertile men with impaired pituitary function.

See also:– FSH, LH, PMHG, PMSG.

HEMICHOLINIUM-3

Competes with choline for transport into cholinergic nerves. Hence transmitter (**ACETYLCHOLINE**) levels are depleted and transmission fails.

Close structural analogue of choline.

Uses:– experimental tool

HEPARIN

Enhances the formation of inactive complexes between the cofactor plasma antithrombin and the clotting factors thrombin, Factors IX and X.

Polyacidic sulphated mucopolysaccharide; hence not active after oral administration. Naturally occurring in liver, lungs and especially Mast cells, where it is stored in complex with amphoteric protein and basic histamine and 5-HT.

Uses:– i) treatment of thrombotic disorders, e.g. deep-vein thromboses, post-operative thrombosis, disseminated coagulation and prophylactically during cardiac surgery or renal dialysis

ii) anti-coagulant added to specimen tubes for blood samples.

Precautions:– i) excessive doses can lead to spontaneous haemorrhage – heparin can be rapidly inactivated by the administration of the basic **PROTAMINE SULPHATE**, which forms a stable salt

ii) commercially available preparations are of non-human animal origin and may give rise to hyper sensitivity reactions, e.g. anaphylaxis.

See also:– warfarin.

HEROIN
See **DIAMORPHINE**.

HEXAMETHONIUM

Competitive antagonist at nicotinic cholinoceptors of autonomic ganglia.
Bisquaternary.

Uses:– experimental tool only.

See also:– trimetaphan.

HISTAMINE

Agonist at H_1 and H_2 histamine receptors.

Derived from amino acid histidine (decarboxylation). Mediator in allergic and inflammatory conditions. Stored in complex with amphoteric protein and **HEPARIN** in Mast cells.

Uses:– experimental tool only.

HOMATROPINE

As **ATROPINE** but shorter duration of action.

Uses:– i) as **ATROPINE**
ii) as cycloplegic to allow optical prescribing by refraction in young children (given as eye-drops).

5-HT (SEROTONIN)

Normal transmitter in certain central neurones. Also stored in platelets and enterochromaffin cells of GI tract. Agonist at 5- HT_1, $5\text{-}HT_2$ and $5\text{-}HT_3$ receptors.

Highly polar, derived from the amino acid tryptophan (hydroxylation then decarboxylation).

Uses:– experimental tool only.

HYDRALAZINE

Vasodilator. Mechanism of action unknown.

Metabolised by acetylation.

Uses:– i) treatment of mild to moderate hypertension, in association with diuretics or antagonists at β-adrenoceptors
ii) treatment of congestive cardiac failure.

Precautions:– i) slow acetylators need smaller doses
ii) may cause systemic lupus erythematosus-reversible.

HYDROCORTISONE

One of the hormones produced by the adrenal cortex. Possesses both glucocorticoid and mineralocorticoid properties.

Highly lipid soluble, but water soluble esters are available for intravenous injection. Around 90% bound to protein (either the corticosteroid binding globulin - high affinity, low capacity – or plama albumin – low affinity, high capacity). Rapidly inactivated (half-life about 1.5 h) by reduction (4,5 double bond) and excreted largely in conjugated form.

Uses:– i) replacement therapy in adrenocortical insufficiency
ii) treatment of allergic and inflammatory conditions.

Precautions:– i) inhibits production of ACTH from pituitary – hence adrenocortical insufficiency if withdrawn
ii) increased risk of peptic ulcer formation
iii) suppression of immune system may increase risk of infection.

5-HYDROXYTRYPTAMINE (SEROTONIN)
See 5-HT.

HYDROXYZINE
As **CHLORPHENIRAMINE** but more potent sedative and antagonist at muscarinic cholinoceptors.

Highly lipid soluble.

Uses:– i) as **CHLORPHENIRAMINE**
ii) anxiolytic
iii) premedication.

Precautions:– marked sedation expected.

HYOSCINE
As **ATROPINE** but more lipid soluble. Also causes sedation & amnesia.

Uses:– i) as **ATROPINE** – may be preferred for premedication because of sedative properties
ii) prophylactic treatment of motion sickness.

I

IBUPROFEN
As **ASPIRIN** but less risk of precipitating Reye's syndrome.

IMIPRAMINE
Inhibitor of **NORADRENALINE** uptake (Uptake$_1$). Also antagonist at muscarinic cholinoceptors and sedative.

Member of the "tricyclic" group of anti-depressants.

Highly lipid soluble, but approximately 98% protein bound; metabolised (desmethylation) to active **DESIPRAMINE**, so that long duration of action (half life ca. 18 h) is due to combined effects of the two drugs.

Uses:– i) treatment of depressive illness

ii) treatment of nocturnal enuresis in children.

Precautions:– i) note that most of the adverse effects result from extensions of the normal pharmacology, e.g. via augmentation of noradrenergic transmission, potentiation of exogenous sympathomimetics, interference with cholinergic transmission
ii) additive effect with other CNS depressants.

IMPROMIDINE

Agonist at histamine receptors; highly selective for H_2 rather than H_1 (10000-fold).

Uses:– experimental tool only.

INDAPAMIDE

As **BENDROFLUAZIDE**.
Structure related to the thiazides.

INDOMETHACIN

As **ASPIRIN** but less risk of precipitating Reye's syndrome.

INDORAMIN

As **PRAZOSIN**.

INSULIN

Hypoglycaemic hormone produced by the B-cells of the pancreatic Islets of Langerhans. Structurally a small protein with a molecular weight of close to 6000 composed of two peptide chains, one of 21 residues, the other of 30 residues joined by two disulphide bonds.

Available in a number of different forms which release active insulin at different rates after injection:–

Short acting (ca. 8 h)
Acid insulin
Neutral insulin
Medium-long acting (ca. 12-24 h)
Biphasic insulin (twice daily)
Amorphous zinc insulin (twice daily)
Isophane insulin (twice daily)
Crystalline zinc insulin (once or twice daily)
Protamine zinc insulin (once daily)

Mainly prepared by extraction from slaughterhouse derived pancreases (pig or ox), but human sequence insulin is now becoming available, produced using recombinant gene technology.

IPRATROPIUM BROMIDE

As **ATROPINE** but quaternary.

Uses:– as aerosol to dilate airways in obstructive airway disease, esp. chronic bronchitis.

IPRONIAZID

As **PHENELZINE**.

ISOCARBOXAZID

Hydrazine type of monoamine oxidase inhibitor; not selective for isozyme A or B.

Highly lipid soluble.

Uses:– antidepressant.

Precautions:– May precipitate hypertensive episodes in response to food containing tyramine, e.g. cheeses, autolysed yeast, pickled herrings, chianti.

See also:– phenelzine, selegiline, tranylcypromine.

ISONIAZID

Anti-tubercular drug; mechanism of action unknown. Also inhibitor of monoamine oxidase.

Metabolised mainly by acetylation.

Uses:– treatment of tuberculosis (as part of "triple therapy").

Precautions:– i) reduce dose in slow acetylators
ii) risk of interaction with dietary amines and sympathomimetics
iii) hypotensive.

See also:– ethambutol, rifampicin, streptomycin.

ISOPRENALINE

Agonist at β-adrenoceptors. Has no selectivity for bronchial β-adrenoceptors (β_2-) as opposed to cardiac β-adrenoceptors (β_1-).

Substrate for Uptake$_2$ and COMT; resistant to Uptake$_1$ and MAO.

Uses:– bronchodilator in asthma (as aerosol).

Precautions:– now considered obsolete due to risk of cardiac stimulation.

See also:– ephedrine, ipratropium, rimiterol, salbutamol.

ISOSORBIDE NITRATE

As **GLYCERYL TRINITRATE** but more resistant to liver enzymes - hence active after oral administration. Available as either mononitrate or dinitrate; active moiety is the nitrate.

KAINIC ACID

Agonist at glutamate receptors (quisqualate type).

Uses:– experimental tool only.

KALLIDIN

As **BRADYKININ**. Kallidin is lysyl-bradykinin, formed in the same way as and rapidly converted to **BRADYKININ** by plasma aminopeptidase.

KALLIKREIN

Generic name for a family of proteolytic enzymes that convert plasma α_2-globulins (the kininogens) to the active kinins **BRADYKININ** and **KALLIDIN**. Plasma kallikrein circulates as the inactive **PREKALLIK-REIN** which is activated by a variety of circumstances (e.g. contact with wettable surfaces & blood clotting Factor XII).

KANAMYCIN

As **GENTAMICIN** but also active against *Mycobacterium tuberculosis*, but does not have a place in the routine treatment of TB.

See also:– gentamicin, neomycin, streptomycin.

KETAMINE

Non-barbiturate anaesthetic for intravenous administration. Analgesic at sub-anaesthetic doses. Vivid dreams, dysphoria and hallucinations common (possibly via dopamine receptors as prevented by dopamine antagonists, e.g. **CHLORPROMAZINE**); incidence lower in children.

Very short duration of action.

Uses:– induction of anaesthesia.

Precautions:– psychotic effects limit usefulness in adults.

KETANSERIN

Antagonist at $5\text{-}HT_2$ receptors. Also antagonist at α-adrenoceptors, histamine H_1 receptors and dopamine receptors.

Uses:– experimental tool.

KETAZOLAM

As **DIAZEPAM**.

KETOCONAZOLE

As **MICONAZOLE**, but more lipid soluble. Also high risk of inducing fatal liver damage.

KETOPROFEN

As **ASPIRIN**, but less risk of inducing Reye's syndrome.

KETOTIFEN

As **CHLORPHENYRAMINE**. Also reputed to have action like **SODIUM CROMOGLYCATE**.

Uses:– prophylaxis and relief of asthma and hay fever.

Precautions:– **i)** adverse effects due to antagonism at muscarinic cholinoceptors
ii) enough drug can cross blood-brain barrier to produce sedation – hence risk if driving, operating machinery, or taking other sedatives
iii) prophylactic action may take 2 weeks to become established.

L

LABETALOL

Competitive antagonist at both α- and β-adrenoceptors (see **PHENTO-LAMINE** & **PROPRANOLOL**).

Some intrinsic activity at β-adrenoceptors.

High lipid solubility – marked "first-pass" metabolism.

Uses:– effective in lowering BP in essential hypertension and hypertensive crisis.

Precautions:– as **PROPRANOLOL** & **PHENTOLAMINE** (but less reflex tachycardia).

LEPTAZOL

Convulsant – possibly acting as **GABA** antagonist.

Uses:– experimental tool only (screening model for anti-convulsants).

LEUKOTRIENES

Derivatives of **ARACHIDONIC ACID** formed in inflammatory and allergic conditions. **SRSa** (slow reacting substance of anaphylaxis) is a mixture of leukotrienes.

Uses:– experimental tools only.

LEVODOPA (L-DIHYDROXYPHENYLALANINE)

Amino acid precursor of dopamine.

Crosses blood-brain barrier by active uptake.

Uses:– idiopathic Parkinson's disease (less effective in post-encephalitic parkinsonism and inappropriate for treating extra-pyramidal symptoms induced by anti-psychotic dopamine antagonists).

Precautions:– i) unwanted peripheral actions – nausea, vomiting & tachycardia (but these greatly reduced by concurrent administration of peripheral DOPA- decarboxylase inhibitor, e.g. **BENSERAZIDE** &/or selective MAO-B inhibitor, e.g. **SELEGILINE**)
ii) excessive doses may result in involuntary movements & psychoses.

See also:– amantidine, benzhexol, bromocriptine.

LEVORPHANOL

As **METHADONE**. Laevo-isomer of **DEXTRORPHAN**.

LEWISITE

Chemical weapon developed and used in World War I. Both vesicant and toxic by virtue of arsenic contained in structure – dichloro(2-chlorvinyl)arsine.

Antidote developed – British Anti-Lewisite (**BAL**) or **DIMERCAPROL** (chelating agent).

LH (LUTEINISING HORMONE)

Pituitary gonadotrophin responsible for ovulation and conversion of Graaffian follicle into corpus luteum and consequent production of **PROGESTERONE**. In mature males stimulates production of **TESTOSTERONE** by Leydig cells of testes.

See also:– FSH, HCG, HMG, PMSG.

LIGNOCAINE

Na^+ channel blocker – hence local anaesthetic and anti- dysrhythmic.

An amide. Moderately lipid soluble – enters CNS readily.

Uses:– i) infiltration and nerve block local anaesthesia (for infiltration often combined with **NORADRENALINE** or **FELYPRESSIN** to prolong action)
ii) suppression of ventricular dysrhythmias especially after myocardial

infarction.

Precautions:– i) excessive doses may cause convulsions – hence reduce dose in patients with impaired liver function
ii) will exacerbate atrio-ventricular block
iii) will depress myocardial contractility in patients with cardiac failure.

LITHIUM

Inhibitor of inositol monophosphate dephosphorylation. This results in interference with the IP_3 intracellular second messenger system by reducing supplies of inositol for reincorporation into membrane phosphatidyl inositol bisphosphate (PIP_2) stores. Selective for CNS as inositol cannot enter CNS readily; in periphery shortfall of inositol made up for by *de novo* synthesis in liver.

Uses:– prophylactic treatment of manic and depressive illness.

Precautions:– i) very small therapeutic index – exacerbated by low plasma Na^+
ii) long-term use may cause kidney damage.

LORAZEPAM

As **DIAZEPAM**, but shorter half-life (ca. 15 h).

LSD (LYSERGIC ACID DIETHYLAMIDE)

Hallucinogen; agonist at central presynaptic 5-HT receptors, especially those on raphe neurones (and probably dopamine receptors).

Derivative of ergot.

Uses:– no therapeutic usefulness but sometime popular "recreational" drug.

Precautions:– panic episodes ("bad trips") may occur. If severe, neuroleptics, e.g. **CHLORPROMAZINE** will terminate the "trip".

See also:– mescaline, psilocin, psilocybin.

LYPRESSIN

As **ADH**, but slightly more resistant to degradation.

Chemically identical to **ADH** except that Arg in the 8 position is replaced by Lys.

See also:– desmopressin, felypressin, oxytocin.

LYSINE VASOPRESSIN

See **LYPRESSIN**.

MAGNESIUM SULPHATE (EPSOM SALTS)

Osmotic laxative (sulphate ion impermeant).

Uses:– i) rapid bowel evacuation (2 h) in occasional constipation
   ii) correction of magnesium deficiency (in intravenous drip).

McN-A-343

Agonist at muscarinic cholinoceptors. Highly selective for M_1 sub-type.

Uses:– experimental tool.

See also:– bethanechol, pirenzepine.

MECAMYLAMINE

As **HEXAMETHONIUM**.

MECLIZINE (USP)

See **MECLOZINE**.

MECLOFENAMATE

As **ASPIRIN**, but of little if any clinical value.

MECLOFENOXATE

General CNS stimulant (analeptic) – mechanism unknown.

Uses:– pharmacological curiosity.

MECLOZINE

As **CHLORPHENIRAMINE**.

Uses:– treatment of nausea and motion sickness (presumably not by action at dopamine receptors as ineffective in preventing **APOMORPHINE**-induced vomiting).

MEDAZEPAM

Prodrug of **DIAZEPAM**. Also active itself.

MEDROXYPROGESTERONE

As **NORETHISTERONE** but lower androgenic potency as analogue of

naturally occuring **PROGESTERONE** rather than **TESTOSTERONE**.
The ester, medroxyprogesterone acetate, is rapidly metabolised after oral doses ("first-pass" effect), but can be given as a "depot" injection – duration of action up to 6 months.

MEFENAMIC ACID
As **ASPIRIN**, but less risk of inducing Reye's syndrome.

MENOTROPHIN
See **FSH**.

METERGOLINE
As **METHYSERGIDE**.

MEPERIDINE (USP)
See **PETHIDINE**.

MEPYRAMINE
As **CHLORPHENYRAMINE**, but obsolete in therapeutics.

MERCAPTOPURINE
Structural analogue of purines – hence interferes with synthesis of purines and therefore of DNA.

Uses:– maintainance therapy for acute leukaemias.

Precautions:– i) as with all anti-metabolites, adverse effects predictable on the basis of the drug's pharmacology, i.e. interference with rapid cell division
ii) **ALLOPURINOL** inhibits metabolism of mercaptopurine – hence potentiation.

See also:– acyclovir, cytarabine, fluorouracil, idoxuridine, methotrexate, zidovudine.

MESCALINE
Potent hallucinogen.

Structural analogue of **DEXAMPHETAMINE**, but low potency as sympathomimetic. Naturally occurring in South American cactus, *Lophophora williamsi (Anhalonium lewinii)*.

Uses:– sometime ingredient of folk religion in Mexico; also recreational drug.

Precautions:– may cause panic reactions ("bad trips") and possibly may uncover latent psychoses.

See also:– LSD, psilocybin.

MESNA

Selectively reacts with acrolein, metabolite of **CYCLOPHOS-PHAMIDE**, which causes haemorrhagic cystitis.

Moderately polar – active after oral administration, although usually given at first as intravenous infusion together with **CYCLOPHOS-PHAMIDE**.

Uses:– to protect against irritation of bladder during chemotherapy with **CYCLOPHOSPHAMIDE**.

Precautions:– one of the metabolic products of MESNA inactivates cytochrome P_{450} – hence impairs metabolism of self and other drugs.

METARAMINOL

As **NORADRENALINE** but highly selective for α-adrenoceptors. Non-catechol and possesses α-methyl substituent.

METFORMIN

Oral hypoglycaemic agent – possibly acts by promoting uptake of glucose by muscle and/or increasing cell sensitivity to **INSULIN**. Only effective if B-cells producing **INSULIN** – hence ineffective against juvenile onset diabetes.

Chemically a biguanide. Lipid soluble.

Uses:– control of maturity onset diabetes, especially in obese patients who have difficulty in restricting their diets.

Precautions:– i) in patients with impaired buffering capacity, (renal failure), risk of lactic acidosis
ii) often causes anorexia and weight loss.

See also:– tolbutamide.

METHACHOLINE

As **ACETYLCHOLINE** but selective for muscarinic cholinoceptors.

Hydrolysed slower than **ACETYLCHOLINE** as susceptible to acetyl-cholinesterase but β-methyl substituent conveys resistance to butyryl-cholinesterase.

Quaternary.

Uses:– as experimental tool only.

METHADONE

As **MORPHINE** but more lipid soluble and more slowly metabolised.

METHIMAZOLE

Active metabolite of **CARBIMAZOLE**.

METHIONINE

Sulphur containing amino acid.

Uses:– to restore hepatic stores of glutathione in cases of overdose with **PARACETAMOL**.

See also:– acetylcysteine.

METHOTREXATE

Essentially irreversible inhibitor of dihydrofolate hydrogenase (has 100000 times the affinity of natural substrate).

Moderately lipid soluble (absorbed from the GI tract), but excreted largely unchanged by the kidney.

Uses:– treatment of solid tumours and leukaemias; can cure choriocarcinoma.

Precautions:– with most anti-metabolites causes myelosuppression as an extension of desired activity. Recovery can be accelerated by the administration of **FOLINIC ACID** which bypasses the blocked enzyme and allows purine and pyrimidine synthesis to resume.

METHOXAMINE

As **NORADRENALINE**, but selective for α-adrenoceptors. Non-catechol and possesses α-methyl substituent.

Uses:– to elevate blood pressure during general or spinal anaesthesia.

See also:– adrenaline, noradrenaline, phenylephrine.

METHOXYFLURANE

As **HALOTHANE** but more potent analgesic.

Precautions:– usefulness limited by renal toxicity due to release of fluoride ions, especially when renal function already impaired.

METHYLCELLULOSE

Bulk forming laxative.

Uses:– i) treatment of constipation associated with low fibre intake
ii) treatment of diverticular disease.

Precautions:– intestinal obstruction.

METHYLCELLULOSE

Bulk forming laxative.

Uses:– **i)** treatment of constipation associated with low fibre intake **ii)** treatment of diverticular disease.

Precautions:– intestinal obstruction.

METHYLCYSTEINE

As **CARBOCISTEINE**.

METHYLDOPA

Competes with the amino acid DOPA for DOPA-decarboxylase in synthesis of dopamine, noradrenaline & adrenaline. Mechanism of hypotensive action likely two-fold:–

i) depletes transmitter stores in dopaminergic, adrenergic & noradrenergic neurones (main effect via peripheral sympathetic neurones) **ii)** formation of false-transmitter (α-methylnoradrenaline) which is potent agonist at inhibitory presynaptic $α_2$-adrenoceptors in CNS (cf. **CLONIDINE**).

Uses:– treatment of moderate to severe hypertension, esp. if antagonist at β-adrenoceptors contra-indicated.

Precautions:– **i)** may cause sedation & depression **ii)** may cause liver damage on prolonged use **iii)** may sensitize red cells leading to haemolytic anaemia (positive Coomb's test).

METHYLPHENIDATE

As **DEXAMPHETAMINE** and **COCAINE** but not local anaesthetic; structural resemblance to both **COCAINE** and **DEXAMPHETAMINE**.

Uses:– experimental tool only.

α-METHYL TYROSINE

See **METIROSINE**.

METHYLXANTHINES

Group of related drugs that inhibit nucleotide phosphodiesterase. See **THEOPHYLLINE**.

Many from natural sources – **CAFFEINE** in tea, cola nuts and coffee; **THEOBROMINE** in cocoa.

METHYL SALICYLATE

Commonly known as "Oil of Wintergreen". Pharmacology as **ASPIRIN** but far too toxic to be given for systemic use to man.,

Uses:– topically as rubefacient.

METHYSERGIDE

Antagonist at 5-HT$_2$ receptors and partial agonist at 5-HT$_1$ receptors.

Highly lipid soluble; structurally related to the **ERGOT ALKALOIDS**.

Uses:– i) prophylaxis of migraine
ii) to inhibit the excessive gastro-intestinal motility of the carcinoid syndrome; does not prevent the vascular dilatation.

Precautions:– prolonged use causes irreversible retroperitoneal fibrosis. For this reason methysergide is now obsolescent, if not obsolete in therapeutics.

METIROSINE (α-METHYL TYROSINE)

Competes with tyrosine for tyrosine hydroxylase and thereby inhibits synthesis of dopamine, noradrenaline and adrenaline.

Transported across blood–brain barrier like tyrosine.

Uses:– to reduce hypertension and anxiety in phaeochromocytoma.

Precautions:– i) sedation, diarrhoea & extrapyramidal symptoms are unavoidable consequences of the drug's pharmacology
ii) poorly soluble in water therefore crystaluria may develop if fluid intake not maintained.

See also:– benserazide, phenoxybenzamine, phentolamine, propranolol.

METITEPINE

As **METHYSERGIDE**, but less selective.

Uses:– experimental tool only.

METOCLOPRAMIDE

As **CHLORPROMAZINE** but shows some selectivity as an anti-emetic, possibly because less lipid soluble and crosses blood-brain barrier less well (excreted largely unchanged by the kidney). However extra-pyramidal symptoms and hyper-prolactinaemia common.

Uses:– treatment of severe vomiting, especially after cytotoxic drug therapy for neoplastic disease.

Precautions:– adverse effects result from extension of desired pharmacology.

METRONIDAZOLE

Prodrug; active form produced by reduction in anaerobes only (catalysed by ferridoxin) – lethal to *Trichomonas, Entamoeba, Giardia lamblia, Bacteroides, Clostridium difficile, Borrelia vincenti*.

Lipid soluble.

Uses:– treatment of infection with anaerobic bacteria or amoebae.

Precautions:– interferes with **ETHANOL** metabolism (**DISUL-FIRAM**-like).

MIANSERIN

As **IMIPRAMINE**, but may have anti-depressant properties not related to ability to inhibit neuronal uptake of amines. A member of the "quad-ricyclic" group of anti-depressants.

MICONAZOLE

Inhibits formation of ergosterols in the membrane of fungal cells – hence leakage of important intracellular components and cell death.

Moderately polar – absorbed after oral administration but penetrates CNS poorly. After topical administration, absorption slow.

Uses:– i) treatment of localised ringworm (topical application)
ii) treatment of severe infections with *Candida albicans* (topical or systemic)
iii) treatment of systemic fungal infections.

Precautions:– i) miconazole inhibits metabolism of both **PHENY-TOIN** & **WARFARIN**;
ii) may cause liver damage – hence should only be given systemically in cases of severe fungal infection.

See also:– amphotericin, griseofulvin, nystatin, tolnaftate, undecanoates.

MINOCYCLINE

As **TETRACYCLINE** but wider spectrum of activity (includes *Nisseria meningitidis*) and less likely to cause renal damage.

MINOXIDIL

Direct vasodilator – possibly by raising intracellular levels of cyclic GMP. Also stimulates growth of hair (hypertrichosis).

Uses:– i) severe resistant hypertension
ii) recently approved in US as hair restorer.

Precautions:– i) causes severe reflex tachycardia; can be controlled with antagonist at β-adrenoceptors

ii) also causes fluid retention – controlled with a loop diuretic (e.g. **FRUSEMIDE**).

MONOSULFIRAM

Insecticide of unknown mechanism of action. Selectivity due to preferential accumulation by parasite reinforced by topical application (highly water soluble). Also inhibits aldehyde dehydrogenase – close structural analogue **DISULFIRAM**.

Uses:– treatment of scabies infestations.

Precautions:– causes alcohol intolerance (see **DISULFIRAM**).

MORPHINE

Agonist at μ-opioid receptors.

Principal active ingredient of **OPIUM** obtained from the opium poppy *Papaver somniferum*.

Moderately polar – hence slowly absorbed from GI tract. Mainly excreted as a conjugate.

Uses:– i) analgesic (moderate to severe pain, especially after trauma where little inflammation)
ii) anti-tussive
iii) anti-diarrhoeal
iv) recreational drug.

Precautions:– i) tolerance develops rapidly necessitating an increase in the dose
ii) physical dependence also develops – hence withdrawal syndrome
iii) overdose causes death by respiratory depression – commonest cause of death amongst addicts as "street" drug of variable composition.

MUSCARINE

As **ACETYLCHOLINE** but selective for muscarinic cholinoceptors.

Not an ester; quaternary.

Toxic alkaloid constituent of *Amanita muscaria*, the fly agaric mushroom.

Uses:– experimental tool only.

NADOLOL
As **PROPRANOLOL**.

NALOXONE
Competitive antagonist at μ-opioid receptors.

Lipid soluble.

Uses:– treatment of narcotic overdose.

Precautions:– short duration of action (approx. 30 min after clinically effective dose given by injection). Therefore symptoms of overdose may return as naloxone inactivated.

NANDROLONE
As **TESTOSTERONE** but higher potency as anabolic than androgen (but selectivity only 2-3 times).

Alkylated at 17-α-position – hence slow metabolism.

Uses:– i) treatment of breast cancer, especially around the menopause
ii) to improve erythropoiesis in some aplastic anaemias and leukaemias
iii) to increase muscle mass in athletes – effectiveness unproven, but very widely used among "explosive strength event" athletes.

Precautions:– i) virilisation
ii) liver toxicity (cholestatic jaundice).

NAPROXEN
As **ASPIRIN**, but less risk of inducing Reye's syndrome.

NEOMYCIN
As **GENTAMICIN** but too toxic for systemic use.

Uses:– i) suitable for skin infections and for "sterilising" bowel before intestinal surgery. The value of this is unproven
ii) valuable, along with dietary protein restriction, in reducing production of ammonia and amines which cause encephalopathy in liver failure.

See also:– gentamicin, kanamycin, streptomycin.

NEOSTIGMINE
Competitive inhibitor of acetylcholinesterase.

Quaternary.

Uses:– i) treatment of myaesthenia gravis
ii) to accelerate recovery from paralysis due to competitive antagonists at nicotinic cholinoceptors of skeletal neuromuscular junction.

Precautions:– i) adverse effects mainly due to extension of desired pharmacology, primarily parasympathomimesis – generally controllable with antagonists at muscarinic cholinoceptors
ii) stimulation of GI muscarinic cholinoceptors dangerous if GI obstruction present.

See also:– dyflos, ecothiopate, edrophonium, physostigmine.

NICORANDIL

As **CROMOKALIM**, but also smooth muscle relaxant by mechanism other than via K^+ channels – possibly by causing accumulation of cyclic-GMP within smooth muscle cells.

Uses:– experimental hypotensive drug.

NICOTINE

As **ACETYLCHOLINE** but selective for nicotinic cholinoceptors (i.e. ganglia & skeletal neuromuscular junction). Prolonged exposure or high concentrations cause depolarising blockade of transmission &/or receptor desensitisation.

Very lipid soluble.

Active ingredient of tobacco.

Uses:– i) experimental tool
ii) "recreational" drug – smoking, snuff, etc.
iii) in chewing gum as replacement therapy during withdrawal from the tobacco habit.

See also:– DMPP, suxamethonium.

NICOUMALONE

As **WARFARIN**.

NICARDIPINE

As **NIFEDIPINE**.

NIFEDIPINE

As **VERAPAMIL** but lacks activity at those cardiac Ca^{2+} channels involved in the cardiac action potential. Ca^{2+} channels in smooth muscle more sensitive than Ca^{2+} channels in cardiac muscle – hence vasodilatation at doses that have little cardio-depressant activity.

A member of the dihydropyridine group.

Uses:– i) prophylaxis of angina – esp. "variant" or Prinzmetal's type
ii) treatment of Raynaud's syndrome.

Precautions:– adverse effects are largely due to the drug's desired pharmacology, i.e. vasodilatation (flushing, swollen feet, headache, etc.)

NIKETHAMIDE

CNS stimulant.

Uses:– once popular as respiratory stimulant. However stimulant dose too close to convulsant dose to be useful.

See also:– doxapram.

NITRAZEPAM

As **DIAZEPAM**; one of the **BENZODIAZEPINES**. Metabolism largely by acetylation.

Uses:– widely promoted for use as hypnotic. However half-life (ca. 24 h) is similar to the benzodiazepines generally regarded as useful as sedatives or anxiolytics (e.g. **DIAZEPAM**).

Precautions:– i) long half-life implies that "hang over" will occur next day if used as hypnotic
ii) metabolism impaired in genetic slow-acetylators.

NITRENDIPINE

As **NIFEDIPINE**.

NITROPRUSSIDE

See **SODIUM NITROPRUSSIDE**.

NITROUS OXIDE

Gaseous (strictly speaking vaporous) "general anaesthetic". Full surgical anaesthesia & unconsciousness cannot be achieved with 80% N_2O + 20% O_2 at normal pressure. Analgesic (measurable at 20% in inspired air).

Relatively sparingly soluble in plasma therefore rapid induction.

Uses:– i) "carrier" gas during anaesthesia with, e.g. **HALOTHANE** – analgesic action reduces concentration of other anaesthetic needed
ii) analgesic during child-birth (self-administered by means of demand valve)
iii) analgesic for accident victims – carried in ambulances premixed with oxygen 50/50.

Precautions:– i) exposure of patient or theatre staff can cause mega-loblastic anaemia by oxidising cobalt in vitamin B12
ii) analgesia abolished by narcotic antagonists, e.g. **NALOXONE**.

NORADRENALINE

Agonist at α- and β-adrenoceptors (normal transmitter in noradrenergic neurones).

Highly polar. Inactivated by:–
i) uptake
ii) N-oxidation (monoamine oxidase)
iii) O-methylation (catechol-O-methyl transferase)

Uses:– i) as vasoconstrictor to prolong duration of action of local anaesthetics
ii) to elevate blood pressure during anaesthesia.

Precautions:– once popular use to elevate blood pressure in traumatic shock now considered inadvisable as this impairs blood flow to vital organs.

NORDIAZEPAM

Active metabolite of many **BENZODIAZEPINES**, esp. **MEDAZEPAM, DIAZEPAM** & **CHLORAZEPATE**.

Long duration of action (half life ca. 72 h).

NORETHISTERONE

Agonist at progesterone receptors. Close structural analogue of **TESTOSTERONE** – hence also androgenic.

Steroid with 17-α-ethinyl substituent, hence more resistant to hepatic metabolism than, e.g. **MEDROXYPROGESTERONE**.

Uses:– i) as the progestagen in combined type oral contraceptives
ii) as progestagen only contraceptive (either as the acetate taken once a day, or as the enanthate in an oily suspension given as a depot injection – duration of action about 2 months)
iii) treatment of menstrual disorders and endometriosis.

Precautions:– i) virilisation
ii) risk of hepatic damage (cholestatic jaundice).

NORTRYPTYLINE

As **IMIPRAMINE**.

NYSTATIN

As **AMPHOTERICIN**, but too toxic for systemic use. Highly polar – hence selectivity for fungus (esp. *Candida albicans*) enhanced by distribution, e.g. skin or lumen of GI tract.

17-β-OESTRADIOL

As **ETHINYLOESTRADIOL**, but highly lipid soluble and very susceptible to hepatic enzymes; the naturally occurring hormone produced by ovarian follicles.

OMEPRAZOLE

Proton pump (H^+/K^+-ATPase) inhibitor; reversible.

Chemically a substituted benzimidazole; moderately lipid soluble – excreted rapidly from plasma, but has prolonged duration of action as it is selectively accumulated in parietal cells. A single dose may inhibit gastric acid secretion for 1-2 days.

Uses:– i) treatment of peptic ulcers
   ii) control of acid hypersecretion in cases of Zollinger-Ellison syndrome.

Precautions:– new drug.

OPIUM

Mixture of alkaloids obtained from the dried latex of the opium poppy *Papaver somniferum*. Contains mainly **MORPHINE, CODEINE, PAPAVARINE**, together with many components with no or minor pharmacological properties.

Uses:– i) "recreational drug" (illegal)
   ii) analgesic, anti-tussive or constipant – commonly as the hydrochlorides in mixture known as "papavaretum".

Precautions:– as **MORPHINE**.

ORCIPRENALINE

As **ISOPRENALINE**.

OUABAIN

As **DIGOXIN**, but more water soluble.

OXAZEPAM

As **DIAZEPAM**, except shorter half-life (ca. 10 h); one of the active metabolites of many **BENZODIAZEPINES**.

OXYTETRACYCLINE

As **TETRACYCLINE**.

OXOTREMORINE

As **ACETYLCHOLINE** but selective for muscarinic cholinoceptors. Also causes ACh release &/or increased concentrations of ACh in brain – hence tremorigenic.

Very lipid soluble (absorbed through skin).

Uses:– as experimental tool.

See also:– tremorine.

OXPRENOLOL

As **PROPRANOLOL** but marked intrinsic activity.

(The intrinsic activity may render oxprenolol less likely to cause cardiac failure or bronchospasm – not proven.)

OXYPHENBUTAZONE

As **PHENYLBUTAZONE**.

OXYTOCIN

Agonist at oxytocin receptors – natural pituitary hormone involved in the milk let-down reflex, initiation of labour and involution of the uterus after delivery. Although selective for oxytocin receptors, selectivity not high and therefore also stimulates vascular and renal ADH/vasopressin receptors. This forms basis of old bioassay – chicken blood pressure.

Nonapeptide differing from **ADH** only in two locations – Ile instead of Phe at 3 and Leu instead of Arg at 8.

Uses:– i) induction of labour
ii) to facilitate clearance of uterus in incomplete abortion
iii) to limit post-partum haemorrhage
iv) stimulation of milk let-down (administered by nasal insufflation).

Precautions:– i) risk of uterine rupture if obstruction to birth canal or cervix inadequately dilated
ii) other adverse effects due to stimulation of ADH/vasopressin receptors.

PABA (PARA-AMINO BENZOATE)
See p-AMINOBENZOATE.

PANCURONIUM
As **TUBOCURARINE** but does not release histamine and is not antagonist at cholinoceptors of ganglia.

PARACETAMOL
As **ASPIRIN** but apparent selectivity for CNS rather than peripheral cyclo-oxygenase – hence not anti-inflammatory at antipyretic, analgesic doses.

Moderately polar, but very rapidly absorbed from the GI tract. Mainly excreted as glucuronide, but after large doses, conjugation capacity exceeded and the drug is hydroxylated to a highly reactive derivative (N-acetyl-benzoquinoneimine) which reacts with sulphydryl groups – at first stored glutathione. When glutathione stores depleted, the derivative combines with suphydryls on hepatic protein molecules – hence liver necrosis which may be fatal.

Uses:– antipyretic and analgesic for mild, non-inflammatory pain (available without prescription).

Precautions:– liver and kidney damage – risk higher in individuals with low glutathione stores, e.g. children. Antidote is **ACETYLCYSTEINE** or **METHIONINE**.

PARALDEHYDE
As **DIAZEPAM**, but not a benzodiazepine – a cyclic polymer of three acetaldehyde molecules.

Highly lipid soluble. Depolymerised in liver to acetaldehyde, followed by oxidation (as **ETHANOL**).

Uses:– i) treatment of status epilepticus (can be given per rectum)
  ii) to sedate uncooperative agitated patient (e.g. in psychiatic unit).

Precautions:– i) irritant – hence deep intra-muscular injections painful
  ii) can cause skin rashes
  iii) volatile – gives exhaled air an offensive odour.

See also:– barbiturates, benzodiazepines, chloral hydrate, ethanol.

PENICILLAMINE
Chelator of heavy metal ions (esp. lead & copper). Also forms soluble

complex with cystine. Also immunosuppressant, especially in rheumatoid arthritis (perhaps by inhibiting formation of an IgM); action may take 6 months to develop.

Highly lipid soluble – the metal complexes more water soluble, hence excreted by kidney.

Uses:– i) treatment of heavy metal poisoning (copper, lead, mercury)
   ii) removal of excess copper in Wilson's disease
   iii) to dissolve cystine-containing renal stones
   iv) treatment of rheumatoid arthritis (2nd line drug).

Precautions:– i) may cause agranulocytosis or aplastic anaemia – may become irreversible if not detected early
   ii) hypersensitivity may occur (cf. PENICILLIN)
   iii) may cause myaesthenia gravis after prolonged administration
   iv) loss of sense of taste for sweet and salty substances may develop – due to loss of copper; restored by giving small doses of copper.

PENICILLIN

Parent drug for a group of antibiotics. Inhibits formation of bacterial cell wall by inhibiting transpeptidation (cross- linking) – structural analogue of d-alanyl-d-alanine from which insoluble polymer normally formed. Highly selective for bacterial cells as only the l-isomer of alanine utilised in mammalian cells.

Broken down by gastric acid – some varieties resistant, in which case absorption from GI tract can be adequate though incomplete (poorly lipid soluble – hence penetrates CNS poorly). Renal excretion rapid as filtered and secreted by tubule cells; actively removed from CSF by a similar process. Pump can be inhibited by PROBENECID.

Several forms of penicillin available with differing spectra and sensitivities to acid and bacterial β-lactamase:–

   BENZYLPENICILLIN – acid & β-lactamase sensitive; relatively narrow spectrum.

   PHENOXYMETHYLPENICILLIN – acid resistant but sensitive to β-lactamase. Similar spectrum to BENZYLPENICILLIN.

   FLUCLOXACILLIN – resistant to acid & β-lactamase, but similar spectrum to BENZYLPENICILLIN.

   AMPICILLIN – resistant to acid but sensitive to β-lactamase; wider spectrum than BENZYLPENICILLIN.

   AMOXYCILLIN – as AMPICILLIN, but more lipid soluble – hence better absorbed after oral doses. (Also available in a preparation which contains CLAVULINIC ACID, which inhibits β-lactamase and renders the AMOXYCILLIN effective against β-lactamase-producing strains.

   TICARCILLIN – sensitive to acid & β-lactamase, but broad

spectrum. Reserved for use (i.v.) against life-threatening infections with *Pseudomonas aeruginosa*.

Uses:– treatment of bacterial infections (streptococci, pneumo cocci, gonococci, meningococci and actinomycoses, diptheria, gas-gangrene, syphilis, tetanus and yaws. The "broad spectrum" penicillins also active against certain Gram-negative and Gram- positive organisms).

Precautions:– i) some individuals become sensitised to penicillins (previous treatment or in food, e.g. from treated animals). Subsequent exposure causes life-threatening anaphylactic shock. Cross-reactivity with the **CEPHALOSPORINS**, e.g. **CEPHRADINE**
ii) ecology of gut flora disturbed – hence diarrhoea common
iii) may accelerate excretion of oral contraceptive steroids by reducing rate of break down of conjugates by gut bacteria hence interrupting enterohepatic cycling.

PENTAGASTRIN

Synthetic analogue of the C-terminal pentapeptide of **GASTRIN**, the secretogogue transmitter in the stomach.

Uses:– occasionally to test gastric function.

PENTAZOCINE

As **MORPHINE**, but mixed properties – agonist at ⲕ- but antagonist at μ-opioid receptors.

Synthetic non-morphinan.

Precautions:– hallucinations and dysphoria (predictable because an antagonist at μ-receptors).

See also:– pethidine.

PENTOBARBITONE

As **DIAZEPAM**, but chemically a **BARBITURATE**; induces liver enzymes.

Uses:– experimental tool.

PENTOLINIUM

As **HEXAMETHONIUM**.

PENTYLENETETRAZOL (USP)

See **LEPTAZOL**.

PEMOLINE

CNS stimulant of unknown mechanism of action (possibly **DEXAM-**

PHETAMINE-like).

Uses:– experimental tool &/or pharmacological curiosity. (No therapeutic usefulness yet demonstrated.)

PERCHLORATE

See **POTASSIUM PERCHLORATE**.

PETHIDINE

As **MORPHINE**, but chemically a phenylpiperidine (first synthetic narcotic analgesic with structure lacking morphinan ring). Also antagonist at muscarinic cholinoceptors. Metabolite is CNS stimulant, hence risk of hallucinations, dysphoria and convulsions at high doses.

Shorter duration of action than **MORPHINE** (half life ca. 4 h).

Uses:– analgesic during final stages of delivery.

Precautions:– adverse effects largely extensions of main or secondary pharmacology (respiratory depression, dry mouth, convulsions). If sufficient crosses placenta it produces depression of neonate – the "floppy baby" syndrome; improved by narcotic antagonist (e.g. **NALOXONE**).

PHENACETIN

Prodrug of **PARACETAMOL**. Considered too toxic (liver and kidney) for use in man.

PHENACETOPERANE

As **METHYLPHENIDATE**.

PHENAZONE

As **ASPIRIN**, but less risk of inducing Reye's syndrome.

PHENELZINE

Inhibitor of MAO. Hydrazine-like side chain renders inhibition irreversible. Devoid of **DEXAMPHETAMINE**-like actions.

Uses:– treatment of depressive illness.

Precautions:– i) may cause liver damage
ii) potentially serious hypertension may follow ingestion of amine-containing foods (usually **TYRAMINE**) or medicines, e.g. cheeses, autolysed yeast, OTC cold remedies
iii) may cause hypotension (once explointed therapeutically).

See also:– iproniazid, isocarboxazid, selegiline, tranylcypromine.

PHENOBARBITONE

As **DIAZEPAM**, but a **BARBITURATE** – half life ca. 72 h. Physical dependence inescapable on prolonged use.

Powerful enzyme inducer.

Uses:– anticonvulsant. Almost obsolete.

Precautions:– i) enzyme induction interferes with properties of other drugs, and precipitates attacks in patients with acute intermittant porphyria
ii) risk of rebound seizures on withdrawal.

PHENOXYBENZAMINE

Non-competitive antagonist at α-adrenoceptors (also H_1 histamine receptors and muscarinic cholinoceptors); a 2-halo-alkylamine which alkylates receptors (cf. **CYCLOPHOSPHAMIDE**).

Also inhibits noradrenaline $Uptake_1$ & $Uptake_2$ processes.

Uses:– to limit hypertension in phaeochromocytoma esp. in inoperable cases. (**PHENTOLAMINE** may be preferred during surgical removal of such tumours.)

Precautions:– not suitable for routine treatment of hypertension because of excessive reflex tachycardia.

See also:– dibenamine, phentolamine, prazosin, yohimbine.

PHENOXYMETHYLPENICILLIN

As **BENZYLPENICILLIN**, but resistant to gastric acid. However absorbtion variable.

See also:– amoxycillin, ampicillin, clavulinic acid, ticarcillin.

PHENTOLAMINE

Competitive antagonist at α-adrenoceptors.

Uses:– i) to limit hypertension in phaeochromocytoma (either as "cover" during surgical removal or as chronic treatment in inoperable cases)
ii) to treat hypertensive crises due to **CLONIDINE** withdrawal or "cheese reaction" in patients taking MAO-inhibitors (e.g. **PHENELZINE**)
iii) acute cardiac failure.

Note:– usefulness in essential hypertension minimal because of reflex tachycardia (see **PRAZOSIN**).

See also:– phenoxybenzamine, prazosin, yohimbine.

PHENYLBUTAZONE

As **ASPIRIN**, but also uricosuric. Some selectivity for inflammation rather than fever.

Uses:– in-patient treatment of ankylosing spondylitis when other treatments have been unsuccessful.

Precautions:– i) this potent anti-inflammatory and uricosuric drug is no longer available for general use because of the serious adverse effects that it can cause if used without subjecting patients to careful surveillance
ii) risk of agranulocytosis and aplastic anaemia – hence continous assessment of blood status should be made
iii) causes fluid retention which may precipitate cardiac failure in patients with small cardiac reserve.

PHENYLEPHRINE

As **NORADRENALINE** but selective for α_1-adrenoceptors. Not substrate for COMT or MAO or uptake.

Uses:– i) to elevate blood pressure during anaesthesia
ii) to produce mydriasis without cycloplegia (eye-drops)
iii) as nasal decongestant (aerosol or nasal drops).

Precautions:– rebound congestion after prolonged use as nasal decongestant.

See also:– ephedrine, methoxamine, noradrenaline.

PHENYLPROPANOLAMINE

As **EPHEDRINE** but some direct stimulation of α-adrenoceptors and more polar.

Also substrate for MAO.

Uses:– i) nasal decongestant (common in OTC cold remedies)
ii) may reduce incidence of bed-wetting in children
iii) anorectic (effectiveness in weight-loss programmes unsubstantiated).

Precautions:– as ephedrine but smaller risks and less CNS stimulation. Potentiated by MAO-inhibitors (e.g. **PHENELZINE**).

PHENYTOIN

Membrane stabiliser of:–
i) nerves – blocks Na^+ channels & perhaps reduces efflux of K^+ at rest
ii) cardiac cells – increases an outward K^+ current (i_{K1}) and decreases slope of pacemaker potential by decreasing the outward K^+ pacemaker current (i_{K2}).

May also increase brain GABA levels.

Lipid soluble but incompletely absorbed from GI tract. 90% bound to plasma protein. Metabolising enzymes (hepatic hydroxylases) saturate at low plasma concentrations, hence elimination zero order. Weak enzyme inducer.

Uses:– **i)** anti-convulsant
ii) anti-dysrhythmic (ventricular dysrhythmias, paroxysmal atrial flutter/fibrillation, digoxin-induced superventricular dysrhythmias).

Precautions:– **i)** prolonged use may cause gingival hyperplasia, acne & hirsutism
ii) increase in incidence of lip & palate defects in children born to epileptic women taking phenytoin during pregnancy (benefit probably outweighs risk)
iii) metabolism can be induced by barbiturates & other inducers
iv) induces own metabolism & that of other drugs, e.g. oral contraceptives.

See also:– carbamazepine, diazepam, ethosuximide, lignocaine, phenobarbitone, procainamide, sodium valproate.

PHYSOSTIGMINE

As **NEOSTIGMINE**, but tertiary – only combines with anionic site of acetylcholinesterase when ionised (cation).

Active ingredient of Calabar bean (*Physostigma venosum*) of West Africa.

PHYTOMENADIONE

See **VITAMIN K**.

PICROTOXIN

Antagonist at **GABA** receptors.

Occurs naturally in fish berries (seeds of *Anamirta* species).

Uses:– experimental tool.

See also:– bicuculline.

PILOCARPINE

As **ACETYLCHOLINE** but partial agonist & selective for muscarinic cholinoceptors.

Not an ester. Weak base but lipid soluble.

Naturally occuring in *Pilocarpus* spp.

Uses:– miotic (given as eye-drops).

PIMOZIDE

As **CHLORPROMAZINE** but much higher selectivity for dopamine receptors.

A diphenylbutylpiperidine – related chemically to butyrophenones (e.g. **HALOPERIDOL**).

PINACIDIL

As **CROMOKALIM**.

PINDOLOL

As **PROPRANOLOL**, but partial agonist (intrinsic activity ca. 35%).

PIPRADOL

As **METHYLPHENIDATE**.

PIRBUTEROL

As **SALBUTAMOL**.

PIRENZEPINE

As **ATROPINE**, but shows considerable selectivity for M_1 muscarinic cholinoceptors of stomach, (those concerned with gastric acid secretion). Also polar, hence poor penetration of CNS and minimal sedation.

Uses:– to promote healing of peptic ulcers.

See also:– cimetidine, McN-A-343.

PIROXICAM

As **ASPIRIN**, but less risk of inducing Reye's syndrome.

PIZOTIFEN

As **CHLORPHENIRAMINE**. Also antagonist at 5-HT receptors.
Lipid soluble.

Uses:– treatment of migraine.

Precautions:– i) adverse effects largely due to secondary pharmacology, e.g. dry mouth
ii) sedation interferes with ability to operate complex machinery safely.

PIZOTYLINE (USP)

See **PIZOTIFEN**.

PLASMIN

Also known as **FIBRINOLYSIN**. Fibrinolytic enzyme produced from inactive **PLASMINOGEN** (either in plasma or adsorbed onto fibrin) by activators (endogenous tissue-type plasminogen activator or exogenous agents – **UROKINASE** or **STREPTOKINASE**).

PLASMINOGEN

Inactive precursor of **PLASMIN**.

PMHG (POST MENOPAUSAL HUMAN GONADO-TROPHIN)

See **MENOTROPHIN**.

PMSG (PREGNANT MARE'S SERUM GONADO-TROPHIN)

A glycoprotein (MW ca. 30000) synthesised in the uterus and placenta of pregnant mares. Primarily **LH**-like, but also **FSH**-like.

Uses:– experimental tool.

POTASSIUM PERCHLORATE

Inhibitor of iodine uptake by the thyroid.

Uses:– at one time popular second line drug in the treatment of hyperthyroid states, but risk of aplastic anaemia too great.

PRACTOLOL

As **PROPRANOLOL** but:–
    i) marked selectivity for cardiac β-adrenoceptors (β_1)
    ii) some intrinsic activity
    iii) not local anaesthetic
    iv) poorly lipid soluble.

Precautions:– prolonged use can produce damage to cornea and peritoneum or a lupus erythematosus-like condition (the so-called ocular-muco-cutaneous syndrome). There have been deaths. Practolol is no longer available for general use but is still available in injectable form for the treatment of cardiac emergencies.

PRALIDOXIME

Nucleophylic agent (more so than water) which will displace organo-phosphorus cholinesterase inhibitors (e.g. **DYFLOS**) from esteratic site on cholinesterases. Only effective within a few hours of poisoning as enzyme soon undergoes conformational change which results in active centre becoming "hidden" from aqueous phase – hence totally irreversible inhibition.

Uses:– antidote to organophosphorus cholinesterase inhibitors, e.g. nerve gasses in warfare or insecticides (often in self-injecting syringe along with **ATROPINE** & **DIAZEPAM**).

PRAZOSIN

Competitive antagonist at α-adrenoceptors with selectivity for post-synaptic α-adrenoceptors (α_1-) . Hence auto-inhibition via pre-synaptic α-adrenoceptors (α_2-) of noradrenaline release from cardiac sympathetic neurones unimpaired. Thus risk of excessive reflex tachycardia minimal.

Uses:– i) limitation of hypertension in phaeochromocytoma (either as "cover" during surgical removal of tumour or as chronic treatment in inoperable cases)
ii) essential hypertension
iii) cardiac failure.

See also:– phenoxybenzamine, phentolamine, yohimbine.

PREDNISOLONE

Synthetic glucocorticoid (selectivity for gluco- as opposed to mineralo-corticoid properties moderate only – ca. 5-fold).

Highly lipid soluble.

Uses:– i) anti-inflammatory, e.g. in rheumatoid arthritis
ii) treatment of allergic disorders; chronic low doses in severe asthma; large doses to treat allergic emergencies (e.g. status asthmaticus, anaphylactic shock) in conjunction with bronchodilators, e.g. **ADRENALINE, SALBUTAMOL**.

Precautions:– adverse effects exclusively due to normal pharmacology of the drug:–
i) diabetes
ii) osteoporosis
iii) prolonged treatment causes suppresion of production of pituitary **ACTH** and consequent involution of adrenal cortex – hence cortical insufficiency if drug withdrawn rapidly
iv) suppresion of immune system may predispose to infection
v) risk of peptic ulcer formation
vi) mineralocorticoid effects appear at high doses.

See also:– dexamethasone, fludracortisone, hydrocortisone.

PREKALLIKREIN

Inactive precursor of **KALLIKREIN** in the blood.

PRILOCAINE

As **LIGNOCAINE**, but not of value in treatment of cardiac dys-rhythmias.

PRIMAQUINE

Anti-malarial. Prodrug which is activated by the liver. Plasmodium gametocytes and liver-resident forms are deficient in co-factors of the pentose-phosphate pathway, which is normally responsible for generating reduced glutathione. These active derivatives of primaquine can therefore inflict oxidative damage on the parasites – lethal.

Primaquine itself is very lipid soluble; active metabolites much less so.

Uses:– radical cure of benign malaria.

Precautions:– i) because primaquine itself is toxic to host, patient should be well before embarking on a course of treatment, i.e. should have first been made clinically well (**CHLOROQUINE**)
ii) erythrocytes of patients with genetic glucose-6-phosphate dehyd-rogenase deficiency are also susceptible to damage by the active metabolites of primaquine – hence haemolysis and methaemog-lobinaemia.

See also:– quinine.

PROBENECID

Inhibitor of active secreting systems for organic acids across epithelial membranes, e.g. kidney tubule, subarachnoid plexus. Hence substrates for these secreting systems are not transported, e.g. **PENICILLINS** (in-hibition of secretion into renal tubule lumen), uric acid (inhibition of reabsorbtion from lumen of tubules).

Uses:– i) to delay the excretion of **PENICILLINS** (currently minor use)
ii) uricosuric in gout
iii) to hide evidence of drug abuse in athletes subjected to "random" (i.e. notice given) urine tests.

Precautions:– i) when commencing treatment of gout, water intake should be kept high to prevent formation of urate crystals in the kidney
ii) potentiates drugs that are excreted by secretion into tubule.

PROCAINAMIDE

As **QUINIDINE**. Chemically as **PROCAINE**, but ester bond replaced by amide – hence not substrate for esterases.

PROCAINE

As **LIGNOCAINE**. Chemically an ester, hydrolysis of which yields **PABA** – hence renders sulphonamides less effective. Obsolescent local anaesthetic.

PROGESTERONE

Natural progestagenic steroid produced by the corpus luteum of the ovary.

Highly lipid soluble.

Uses:– as **NORETHISTERONE**.

PROLACTIN

Pituitary hormone responsible for development of milk-producing cells of mammary glands. Prolactin releasing cells in pituitary have inhibitory dopaminergic innervation – hence release of prolactin stimulated by dopamine antagonists, e.g. **CHLOPROMAZINE**, and inhibited by dopamine receptor agonists, e.g. **BROMOCRYPTINE**.

Very close homology with growth hormone (both are proteins which exist in two forms – 23000 and 56000 dalton molecular weights).

PROLINTANE

As **PEMOLINE**.

PROMETHAZINE

As **CHLORPHENYRAMINE**. Chemically a phenothiazine.

PROPRANOLOL

Competitive antagonist at β-adrenoceptors. No selectivity for either cardiac (β_1) or airways (β_2-) adrenoceptors. Does not possess intrinsic activity but is a potent local anaesthetic.

Very lipid soluble; a large fraction of an oral dose is metabolised in the liver ("first-pass" effect).

Uses:– i) to increase exercise tolerance in angina
   ii) to control supraventricular dysrhythmias, especially after myocardial infarction (may also limit size of infarct)
   iii) control of tachycardia in thyrotoxicosis
   iv) phaeochromocytoma (either as cardiac "cover" during surgical removal of tumour or as chronic treatment in inoperable cases)
   v) therapy of essential hypertension – mode of action uncertain
   vi) prophylaxis of migraine – mode of action uncertain

vii) anxiety states involving tremor and tachycardia.

Precautions:– i) precipitation of cardiac failure in patients with small cardiac reserves and of bronchoconstriction in asthmatics unavoidable consequences of the drug's pharmacology
ii) can exacerbate Raynaud's syndrome
iii) may cause vivid dreams &/or mild depression &/or lethargy.

See also:– acebutolol, atenolol, labetalol, oxprenolol, practolol, timolol.

PROPYLTHIOURACIL

As **CARBIMAZOLE**, but shorter half-life (ca. 5 h).

PROSTACYCLIN

Cyclic prostaglandin produced from endoperoxide by vascular endothelium; actions (vasodilation, inhibition of platelet aggregation, dilation of bronchi) oppose those of **THROMBOXANE A$_2$**.

Very labile – half life ca. 2 min in blood.

Uses:– experimental tool (under investigation as vasodilator in ischaemic conditions).

PROSTAGLANDINS

Group of 20-carbon unsaturated fatty acids with cyclic head (C8–C12). Formed from tissue (membrane) phospholipids by the action of phospholipase A$_2$ and subsequently cyclo-oxygenase.

Several types; effects mediated through distinct types of receptors, primarily PGE-type and PGF-type.

Naturally occuring PGs very labile in blood. Synthetic derivatives more stable.

PROTAMINE SULPHATE

Low molecular weight strongly basic protein – binds **HEPARIN**.

Uses:– to treat major haemorrhage due to **HEPARIN** overdose.

Precautions:– i) anti-coagulant in own right therefore doses which exceed those needed to bind all the **HEPARIN** will cause bleeding again
ii) sometimes causes vasodilation, but rarely antigenic.

PSILOCIN

As **LSD**. Minor ingredient of "magic mushrooms" of Mexico (*Psilocybe mexicana*).

See also:– mescalin, psilocybin.

PSILOCYBIN

As **LSD**. Major ingredient of "magic mushrooms" of Mexico (*Psilocybe mexicana*).
See also:- mescalin, psilocin.

PYRETHRIN

Insecticide – mechanism of action similar to **DICOPHANE**. Naturally occurring in pyrethrum daisies (*Chrysanthemum cincerariaefolium*) of Southern Africa.

Uses:- treatment of louse infestation.

Precautions:- allergenic (synthetic pyrethrins less so than preparations made from the flowers).

PYRILAMINE (USP)

See **CHLORPHENIRAMINE**.

QUINALBARBITONE

As **DIAZEPAM**, but chemically a **BARBITURATE**. (Half life ca. 48 h).

QUINESTROL

Prodrug of **ETHINYLOESTRADIOL** (O-dealkylated).

Highly lipid soluble; distributes through body fat and slowly released – hence sustained action.

QUINIDINE

As **LIGNOCAINE**; also antagonist at muscarinic cholinoceptors. Very small therapeutic index – suppresses force of contraction of cardiac, skeletal and smooth (vascular) muscle at doses needed to produce impaired Na^+ flux in electrically excitable tissues.

Chemically dextro-rotatory isomer of **QUININE**. Equipotent with **QUININE** as antimalarial.

Uses:- antidysrhythmic (prophylaxis of re-entry extrasystoles).

Precautions:- i) may cause hypersensitivity reaction
  ii) will exacerbate heart block

iii) adverse effects due to action at muscarinic cholinoceptors

iv) causes "cinchonism" (see **QUININE**).

QUININE

As **CHLOROQUINE**. Less potent as antidysrhythmic than **QUINIDINE**.

Precautions:– i) as **QUINIDINE**

ii) prolonged use or high doses can lead to "cinchonism" – tinnitus leading to deafness, disturbed vision, nausea, and reduced force of muscular contraction (smooth & skeletal) – hence hypotension and muscle weakness (and relief of nocturnal cramps).

R

RADIOACTIVE IODINE

See **IODINE**.

RANITIDINE

As **CIMETIDINE**, but more polar and higher selectivity for histamine receptors.

RENIN

Enzyme (MW ca. 40,000) produced by juxtaglomerular apparatus of kidney in response to low plasma Na^+, low pressure or reduced kidney blood flow. Rapidly metabolised by liver (plasma half-life ca. 15 min). Produces **ANGIOTENSIN I** from plasma **ANGIOTENSINOGEN**.

RENNIN

Enzyme produced in stomach, particularly of young animals. Coagulates caseinogen to form casein.

RESERPINE

Depletes adrenergic, noradrenergic, dopaminergic and serotonergic neurones of their transmitter stores by inhibiting vesicular uptake mechanisms.

Highly lipid soluble.

Naturally occurring in climbing shrub (*Rauwolfia serpentina* [Benth]) indigenous to Indian subcontinent.

Uses:– i) pharmacological tool
  ii) to lower blood pressure in severe hypertension resistant to other, safer drugs.

Precautions:– i) depletion of central amine stores can lead to severe, even suicidal, depression
  ii) depletion of central dopamine stores can lead to hyperprolactinaemia, gynaecomastia and galactorrhoea
  iii) depletion of central amine (mainly **DOPAMINE**) stores can lead to extrapyramidal symptoms
  iv) prolonged use by women may cause breast cancer.

See also:– tetrabenazine.

RIFAMPICIN

Inhibits RNA-polymerase. Selective for micro-organisms because it has higher affinity for the enzyme in bacteria than that in mammalian cells.

Moderate lipid solubility. Rapidly secreted in bile – hence enterohepatic circulation. Deacetylated in liver – deacetylated drug retains antibacterial activity and also secreted in bile, though reabsorption from gut impaired. Very powerful inducer of hepatic enzymes.

Uses:– reserved for the treatment of tuberculosis (constituent of "triple therapy").

Precautions:– i) plasma levels may become very high in patients with hepatic failure unless dose reduced
  ii) colours urine, sweat, saliva, etc., red (will also stain soft contact lenses)
  iii) commonly causes GI disturbances, 'flu-like symptoms, rashes, blood dyscrasias
  iv) reduces plasma levels of other drugs metabolised in liver; on cessation of therapy, doses of other drugs will need readjusting as enzyme induction fades.

See also:– ethambutol, isoniazid, streptomycin.

RIMITEROL

As **SALBUTAMOL**, but shorter duration of action

RITODRINE

As **SALBUTAMOL** – popular mainly as intravenous infusion to delay premature labour.

SALBUTAMOL

As **ISOPRENALINE** but selective for airways, blood vessels, uterus & skeletal muscle (tremor) via β_2-adrenoceptors.

Resistant to COMT, MAO, Uptake$_1$ & Uptake$_2$. Intermediate lipid solubility.

Uses:– **i)** bronchodilation in asthma (aerosol or tablets)
   ii) to delay premature labour.

Precautions:– excessive doses (especially oral) may cause potentially dangerous cardiac stimulation, although risk much less than with nonselective bronchodilators.

See also:– adrenaline, ephedrine, fenoterol, isoprenaline, pirbuterol, rimiterol, terbutaline.

SALCATONIN

Synthetic salmon **CALCITONIN**. Less immunogenic than **CALCITONIN** extracted from pigs' parathyroid glands.

SALICYLIC ACID

Keratolytic.

Uses:– topically to increase rate of loss of surface keratin in hyperkeratotic conditions.

Precautions:– systemic toxicity may develop after prolonged usage on large surface area or if applied to broken skin or weeping lesions.

SARALASIN

Partial agonist at angiotensin receptors; intrinsic activity very low.

Close structural analogue of **ANGIOTENSIN II** – Asp at position 1 replaced with Sar, Ileu at 5 with Val and Phe at 8 with Ala.

Uses:– experimental tool – under investigation for use in man as hypotensive agent.

SAXITOXIN (STX)

As **TETRODOTOXIN**. Synthesised by marine dinoflagellates *Gonyaulax catenella* & *G. tamerensis*. These organisms are responsible for "red tides" and they are accumulated by filter feeders such as bivalves (oysters, mussels, clams, etc.). Shellfish then poisonous to man leading to outbreaks of paralytic shellfish poisoning.

Uses: – experimental tool; also candidate for chemical warfare as extraordinary potency (LD50 in mice ca. 10 micrograms).

SELEGILINE

Inhibitor of MAO – irreversible, "suicide" inhibitor, selective for MAO-B isozyme.

Uses: – adjunct to **LEVODOPA** in treatment of Parkinson's disease.

Note: – does not produce "cheese reaction", cf. **PHENELZINE**.

SEROTONIN

See **5-HT**.

SODIUM AUROTHIOMALATE

Suppresses inflammation and may slow degenerative changes in rheumatoid arthritis. Mechanism of action unknown – possibly by inhibiting the activity of mononuclear phagocytes of the immune system.

Very polar – hence must be injected (deep intra-muscular). Gold concentrates in joint cavities and may be excreted for many months after treatment stopped.

Uses: – treatment of rapidly advancing rheumatoid arthritis that fails to respond to **ASPIRIN**-like drugs. In many cases it will stop the advance of the disease process.

Precautions: – i) treatment with gold salts will not restore damage that has already occurred to joints
ii) lesions of skin and mucous membranes common
iii) kidney damage may occur – appears as proteinuria
iv) blood dyscrasias common – treatment should be accompanied by regular blood tests and should be stopped if abnormalities appear
v) **DIMERCAPROL** chelates gold.

SODIUM CROMOGLYCATE

Prevents Mast cell degranulation in response to antigen binding to cell surface IgEs (possibly limits availability of intracellular Ca^{2+} ions).

Poorly absorbed and susceptible to degradation, hence active only as inhaled aerosol or as eye- or nose-drops.

Uses: – prophylaxis of asthma or hay-fever.

SODIUM NITROPRUSSIDE

Vasodilator (possibly acting via cyclic GMP). Active moeity is thiocyanate produced in the liver from cyanide ions which are released when ferrous ions removed by sulphydryl groups in erythrocytes.

Highly polar – hence must be injected. Solution must be freshly prepared and is light sensitive.

Uses:– (**Note**: in all instances sodium nitroprusside is infused until the desired blood pressure is obtained. If too much given, the thiocyanate ion can be removed by renal dialysis.)
  i) treatment of hypertensive crises
  ii) treatment of congestive cardiac failure.

Precautions:– i) adverse effects largely due to excessive vasodilatation
  ii) high blood concentrations can impair uptake of iodine by thyroid.

See also:– diazoxide, glyceryl trinitrate, hydralazine.

SODIUM VALPROATE

Inhibitor of **GABA** transaminase.

Uses:– treatment of epilepsy, especially effective against absence attacks in children

Precautions:– i) occasionally causes GI disturbances and heartburn
  ii) causes hair loss and weight gain in children
  iii) may cause thrombocytopaenia
  iv) it has been suggested that it may predispose to neural tube defects if taken during pregnancy
  v) small risk of hepatic impairment.

SOMATOSTATIN (GROWTH HORMONE RELEASE INHIBITING FACTOR)

Endogenous peptide transmitter involved in the regulation of **GROWTH HORMONE** release. Also involved in regulation of blood glucose concentration; somatostatin inhibits secretion of both **INSULIN** and **GLUCAGON** and secretion of somatostatin is stimulated by **GLUCAGON**.

Uses:– experimental tool.

SOMATOTROPHIN

See **GROWTH HORMONE**.

SOMATREM

Human sequence **GROWTH HORMONE** prepared by recombinant gene technology. Preferred to extracted **GROWTH HORMONE** for therapy.

Polypeptide – hence must be injected.

Uses:– treatment of short stature due to pituitary insufficiency.

Precautions:– once epiphyses have closed, the hormone should not be given.

SOTALOL

As **PROPRANOLOL**, but highly polar.

SPIPERONE

As **CHLOPROMAZINE**, but more selective for dopamine receptors. Chemically a butyrophenone.

SPIRONOLACTONE

Antagonist of **ALDOSTERONE** – competitive. Selectivity moderate – interacts with other steroid receptors at doses similar to those needed therapeutically.

Uses:– i) diuretic (to reduce oedema in cirrhotic liver failure, in treatment of congestive cardiac failure & hypertension)
ii) treatment of primary aldosteronism
iii) in conjunction with thiazide diuretic (e.g. **BENDRO-FLUAZIDE**) to limit of loss of K^+.

Precautions:– i) K^+ conserving action may become dangerous in patients with hyperkalaemia
ii) may cause gynaecomastia and other disturbances of endocrine function.

SPIROPERIDOL (USP)

See **SPIPERONE**.

SRSa (SLOW REACTING SUBSTANCE OF ANAPHYLAXIS)

Mixture of mediators released during allergic reactions. Composed mainly of **LEUKOTRIENES**.

STANOZOLOL

As **TESTOSTERONE**, but selective for anabolic receptors rather than androgenic receptors (selectivity only 2-3 fold).

Lipid soluble. Alkylation at 17-α-position retards metabolism, but can result in cholestatic jaundice.

Uses:– i) to encourage protein synthesis after major surgery or debilitating disease
ii) widely used by athletes in "explosive strength" events. Value unproven.

Precautions:– small therapeutic index implies that androgenic effects inevitable – hence virilisation in females, suppression of sperm formation and reduction in size of testes in males (post-pubertal).

STILBOESTROL

As **OESTRADIOL**, but synthetic non-steroid. Suspected of being carcinogenic (perhaps in women whose mothers took the drug during pregnancy) – hence reserved for use in post-menopausal breast cancer or prostatic cancer.

STREPTOKINASE

Activator of **PLASMINOGEN**. Protein (non-enzyme) produced by group A β-haemolytic streptococci.

Uses:– in emergencies to lyse life-threatening deep vein thromboses and pulmonary emboli.

Precautions:– allergenic, especially shortly after recovery from streptococcal infection.

STREPTOMYCIN

As **GENTAMICIN** but also active against *Mycobacterium tuberculosis*. Also antagonist at nicotinic cholinoceptors of skeletal muscle end plates (cf. **TUBOCURARINE**).

Precautions:– i) use reserved for the treatment of tuberculosis
ii) can cause muscle weakness and increases degree of paralysis induced by competitive nicotinic antagonists.

See also:– ethambutol, gentamicin, isoniazid, kanamycin, neomycin, rifampicin.

STRYCHNINE

Antagonist at **GLYCINE** receptors, e.g. on α-motorneurone; hence feedback inhibition via Renshaw cell prevented and disinhibition results in spasm of skeletal muscle and death by respiratory paralysis and exhaustion.

Uses:– i) one time use in "tonics" discredited
ii) vermicide – especially for carnivores; meat bait injected with small amounts of strychnine.

SUBSTANCE P

Polypeptide (11 amino acid residues) transmitter in brain and nerves (especially sensory afferents).

SUCCINYL DICHOLINE (USP)
See **SUXAMETHONIUM**.

SULINDAC
As **ASPIRIN**, but less risk of inducing Reye's syndrome.

SULPHAMETHIZOLE
Inhibitor of dihydrofolate synthetase as close structural analogue of **PABA** – hence bacteriostatic as bacteria impermeable to dihydrofolate (folic acid) in environment and must therefore synthesise it. Chemically a **SULPHONAMIDE**.

Moderately polar (but well absorbed from gut) – hence excreted rapidly by kidney and reaches high concentrations in urine.

Uses:– treatment of urinary tract infections.

Precautions:– use should be avoided in conjunction with anti-bacterial agents that act on the rapidly growing phase of the cell cycle as mutually inhibitory.

SULPHAMETHOXAZOLE
A **SULPHONAMIDE**. Available as a mixture with **TRIMETHOPRIM** as **CO-TRIMOXAZOLE** (5 parts to one of **TRIMETHOPRIM**). This mixture is synergistic because it produces "sequential blockade" of the folate pathway and may be more effective than either of the ingredients alone and less likely to allow the development of resistant strains.

SULPHAPYRIDINE
Derived from **SULPHASALAZINE** by bacterial deconjugation in the GI tract. Probably not responsible for the therapeutic action of the parent drug.

Polar, but sparsely water soluble. Absorbed from GI tract and excreted by the kidneys.

SULPHASALAZINE
Anti-inflammatory agent effective in colon against ulcerative colitis. Chemically a highly polar **SULPHONAMIDE** which is degraded by gut flora to **SULPHAPYRIDINE**, which is absorbed and excreted in urine, and **5-AMINOSALICYLATE**, which is the active anti-inflammatory agent.

Precautions:– i) the metabolite **SULPHAPYRIDINE** is sparsely water soluble hence crystalluria may develop if water intake low

ii) blood levels of **SULPHAPYRIDINE** likely to rise dangerously high in patients with impaired renal or liver function or in slow acetylators

iii) may precipitate haemolysis in patients with glucose-6-phosphate dehydrogenase deficiency.

SULPHONAMIDES

Group of anti-bacterial agents that are close structural analogues of **p-AMINOBENZOATE**, the precursor from which many bacteria synthesise dihydrofolate. Selectivity relies on the fact that mammalian cells can absorb dihydrofolate, whereas bacterial cells are impermeant and need to synthesise it.

Because cells have stores of the intermediates used to synthesise purines and pyrimidines, there is a lag between inhibiting synthesis of dihydrofolate and failure of growth and replication.

See also:– sulphones.

SULPHONES

As **SULPHONAMIDES**, but with some selectivity for *Mycobacterium leprae* (see **DAPSONE**).

SULPIRIDE

As **CHLORPROMAZINE**, but more selective for dopamine receptors. Close structural analogue of **METOCLOPRAMIDE**, but higher lipid solubility.

SUXAMETHONIUM

As **ACETYLCHOLINE** but selective for nicotinic cholinoceptors of skeletal muscle. High concentrations cause depolarising blockade of transmission.

Quaternary. Double ester, susceptible to butyrylcholinesterase but resistant to acetylcholinesterase.

Uses:– as muscle relaxant for short procedures, especially intubation, ECT & orthopaedic manipulation.

Precautions:– **i)** approximately 1 in 2500 individuals have a genetically determined atypical form of butyrylcholinesterase. Consequently suxamethonium causes prolonged apnoea (homozygotes). Heterozygotes (ca. 4%) hydrolyse the suxamethonium at an intermediate rate

ii) cholinesterase inhibitors (e.g. **NEOSTIGMINE**) increase degree of and prolong paralysis by retarding hydrolysis

iii) may precipitate malignant hyperthermia in genetically predisposed individuals (see **DANTROLENE** for treatment).

TAMOXIFEN

As **CLOMIPHENE**, but less intrisic activity.

Uses:– as **CLOMIPHENE**, but also useful to treat hormone dependent cancers esp. breast cancer in post menopausal women.

T.E.A. (TETRAETHYLAMMONIUM)

Competitive antagonist at nicotinic cholinoceptors of ganglia. Also blocks K^+ channels.

Quaternary.

Uses:– experimental tool only.

TEMAZEPAM

As **DIAZEPAM**, but shorter half life (ca. 12 h).

TERBUTALINE

As **SALBUTAMOL**.

TERFENADINE

As **CHLORPHENIRAMINE**, but highly polar – hence minimal CNS effects.

TERLIPRESSIN

As **VASOPRESSIN**; synthetic analogue.

TESTOSTERONE

Agonist at androgen and anabolic receptors; the natural male hormone produced by Leydig cells of testes.

Highly lipid soluble steroid – rapidly metabolised; converted to **5-α-DIHYDROTESTOSTERONE** (more potent) in target tissues; available in form suitable for depot injection for prolonged action or as several esters, e.g. enanthate, undecanoate, propionate, etc. which have longer half lives.

Uses:– replacement therapy in hypogonadism.

Precautions:– i) hastens closure of epiphyses – hence can lead to short stature if treatment started too early

ii) accelerates the growth of male hormone dependent tumours,

e.g. prostatic carcinomas
    iii) virilises foetus if given to pregnant woman carrying female foetus.

See also:– cyproterone, stanozolol.

TETRABENAZINE

As **RESERPINE**, but selective for dopaminergic neurones – hence does not cause depression.

Uses:– to control athetoid movements in Huntington's chorea.

TETRACOSACTRIN

Agonist at corticotrophin receptors. Synthetic analogue of first 24 residues of **ACTH**.

Half-life short (peptide), but depot preparations available (zinc complex).

Uses:– i) to test competence of adreno-hypophyseal axis; if adrenal insufficiency is due to pituitary failure, tetracosactrin will induce rise in urinary levels of steroid metabolites
    ii) replacement therapy in patients with anterior pituitary failure, especially children in whom corticosteroids may stunt growth
    iii) instead of corticosteroids in children for treatment of severe inflammatory or allergic diseases.

Precautions:– although tetracosactrin does not cause involution of the adrenals as do the corticoids, it can stimulate overproduction of cortical hormones leading to Cushing's syndrome, peptic ulceration, psychosis, hypertension, etc. Probably also stunts growth in children.

TETRACYCLINE

Broad spectrum antibiotic (Gram positive and negative bacteria, rickettsiae, mycoplasma, chlamydia & some amoebae). Inhibits protein synthesis by binding to 30S subunits of ribosomes. Selective for micro-organisms because of active accumulation.

Intermediate lipid solubility. Chelates metal ions from diet – complex cannot cross intestinal epithelium (e.g. Ca^{2+} from milk, antacids; Fe^{2+} from iron tablets; Al^{3+} from antacids; Mg^{2+} from antacids, Epsom salts, etc.).

Uses:– treatment of Chlamydial infections (trachoma, psittacosis, urethritis, lymphogranuloma venereum), rickettsia (Q-fever), mycoplasm (respiratory & genito-urinary) and brucellosis.

Precautions:– i) chelates Ca^{2+} & therefore stains growing teeth (under 12 years) and bones
    ii) occasionally causes photosensitivity
    iii) occasionally causes hepatic & renal damage.

TETRAETHYLAMMONIUM
See **TEA**.

TETRAMETHYLAMMONIUM
See **TMA**.

TETRODOTOXIN (TTX)
Blocks Na^+ channels (i.e. "membrane stabiliser").

Very rapidly absorbed and distributed.

Occurs in nature in tissues of:–
   i) fish of the *Tetraodontidae* (Puffer fish or Fugu)
   ii) salamanders of the west coast area of N.America.

Uses:– experimental tool only.

See also:– lignocaine, saxitoxin.

Note:– on a molar basis **TTX** approximately 100,000 times more potent than **COCAINE**.

THEOBROMINE
As **CAFFEINE**; naturally occurring in cocoa and chocolate.

THEOPHYLLINE
As **CAFFEINE**.

Forms water-soluble complex with **ETHYLENEDIAMINE** known as **AMINOPHYLLINE**.

Uses:– **i)** bronchodilator in reversible obstructive airway disease (asthma), either oral in mild to moderate cases or intravenous for severe attacks (status asthmaticus)
   ii) left ventricular failure.

Precautions:– **i)** headache, palpitations, GI disturbance, insomnia
   ii) intramuscular injections should not be used as painful.

See also:– caffeine, theobromine.

THIOPENTONE
As **DIAZEPAM**, but much shorter half-life (ca. 6 h). Chemically a **BARBITURATE**.

Uses:– by rapid intravenous injection to induce anaesthesia (onset of anaesthesia rapid – vein to brain circulation time; effect terminated by redistribution into poorly perfused fat deposits).

Precautions:– **i)** hyperalgesic

ii) irritant – hence causes pain and necrosis if injected into tissue or artery rather than vein.

THROMBOXANES

Group of mediators formed from cell (membrane) phospholipid by action of phospholipase A_2, followed by cyclo-oxygenase and thromboxane synthetase (pathway in parallel with **PROSTAGLANDIN** and **PROST-ACYCLIN** formation). Actions essentially opposite to those of **PROST-ACYCLIN** i.e. vasoconstriction, cause aggregation of platelets and constriction of bronchi.

Very labile – half life in blood ca. 30 s.

Uses:– experimental tools.

THYROXINE (SODIUM) (T4)

Thyroid hormone.

Uses:– replacement therapy in hypothyroidisms.

Precautions:– excessive doses induce hyperthyroid state – potentially dangerous if pre-existing heart disease or hypertension.

TICARCILLIN

As **BENZYLPENICILLIN**, but wider spectrum. Reserved for the treatment of life-threatening infections with *Pseudomonas aeruginosa*.

TIMOLOL

As **PROPRANOLOL**.

Uses:– as **PROPRANOLOL** but also available in eyedrop form – reduces rate of aqueous humour production in glaucoma.

Precautions:– very lipid soluble therefore can produce systemic effects (e.g. bronchoconstriction) when instilled into the eye. Deaths have occurred.

TMA (TETRAMETHYLAMMONIUM)

Agonist at nicotinic cholinoceptors of ganglia.

Quaternary.

Uses:– experimental tool only.

See also:– DMPP, hexamethonium, nicotine.

TOLAZAMIDE

As **TOLBUTAMIDE**.

TOLBUTAMIDE

Enhances residual **INSULIN** secretion in maturity onset diabetes.

Chemically substituted sulphonylurea – moderate lipid solubility. Metabolised by oxidation; half life ca. 6 h.

Uses:– hypoglycaemic in maturity onset diabetes.

Precautions:– i) hypoglycaemia is a predictable consequence of overdose, impaired metabolism or inadequate calorie intake
ii) occasionally causes hypersensitivity reaction resulting in aplastic anaemia or agranulocytosis.

See also:– insulin, metformin.

TOLMETIN

As **ASPIRIN**, but less risk of inducing Reye's syndrome.

TOLNAFTATE

Fungicidal agent – effective against dermatophytes, e.g. *Tinea pedis* (athletes' foot). Mechanism of action uncertain – possibly similar to the imidazole derivatives (see **MICONAZOLE**).

Polar – hence not absorbed from skin.

Uses:– treatment of fungal infections of the skin.

See also:– griseofulvin, undecanoates.

TRANEXAMIC ACID

As **AMINOCAPROIC ACID** (structural analogue).

TRANYLCYPROMINE

Competitive inhibitor of MAO. Some stimulation of CNS, cf. **DEXAMPHETAMINE**.

Uses:– treatment of depressive illness.

Precautions:– potentially serious hypertension may follow ingestion of amine-containing foods (usually **TYRAMINE**) or medicines, e.g. cheese, autolysed yeast extracts, OTC cold remedies.

See also:– phenelzine, selegiline.

TREMORINE

Prodrug of **OXOTREMORINE** – oxidised by SER in liver.

TRIAMTERINE

As **AMILORIDE**.

TRIAZOLAM

As **DIAZEPAM**, but much shorter half life (ca. 2 h). Chemically a **BENZODIAZEPINE**.

TRICHLOROETHANOL

Active metabolite of **CHLORAL HYDRATE**.

TRICLOFOS

As **CHLORAL HYDRATE**. Chemically the monosodium salt of the phosphate ester of **TRICHLOROETHANOL**, the active metabolite of **CHLORAL HYDRATE**. More palatable and less irritant than **CHLORAL HYDRATE**.

TRIETHYLCHOLINE

Close structural analogue of choline, the normal precursor of **ACETYL-CHOLINE**. Handled by cholinergic neurones exactly as choline and incorporated into the false transmitter **ACETYLTRIETHYLCHOLINE**, stored in vesicles and released in place of **ACETYLCHOLINE**.

Uses:– experimental tool only.

TRIFLUOPERAZINE

As **CHLORPROMAZINE**.

TRIMETAPHAN

As **HEXAMETHONIUM**.

Not quaternary, but highly polar as structure includes a protonated sulphur atom.

Uses:– to induce hypotension during surgery.

Precautions:– adverse effects are predictable results of the drug's pharmacology.

See also:– mecamylamine, pentolinium, d-tubocurarine.

TRIMETHOPRIM

Structural analogue of dihydrofolate which inhibits DHF hydrogenase of bacteria causing cell growth and replication to cease. Selective for bacteria because it has much higher affinity for bacterial DHF hydrogenase than for the mammalian enzyme.

Moderate lipid solubility – well absorbed but excreted largely in urine by filtration .

Uses:– treatment of urinary tract and respiratory infections.

Precautions:– i) despite selectivity for bacterial form of DHF hydrogenase, folate deficiency may develop on long term therapy, leading to anaemia

ii) in kidney failure, blood concentrations may rise unless dose reduced.

Note:– available in a mixture with **SULPHAMETHOXAZOLE** (5 parts to 1 part of trimethoprim) known as **CO-TRIMOXAZOLE**. This mixture produces "sequential blockade" of the folate pathway and may be more effective in certain cases and less likely to allow the development of resistant strains.

TRIPELENNAMINE

As **CHLOPHENIRAMINE**.

TROPICAMIDE

As **ATROPINE** but very short duration of action.

Uses:– exclusively as mydriatic for diagnostic purposes (given as eyedrops; if dose small enough, adequate mydriasis possible with little or no cycloplegia).

d-TUBOCURARINE

Competitive antagonist at nicotinic cholinoceptors of skeletal muscle. Also at ganglia, but less potent.

Quaternary hence basic.

Uses:– to produce muscle paralysis for surgery.

Precautions:– i) can cause histamine release (because basic) leading to a rash

ii) patients must be artificially ventilated; cholinesterase inhibitors (e.g. **NEOSTIGMINE**) decrease degree of and shorten paralysis by raising ACh concentration at neuromuscular junctions

iii) additive with muscle relaxing general anaesthetics (**ETHER, ENFLURANE, METHOXYFLURANE, HALOTHANE**) and aminoglycoside antibiotics (**GENTAMICIN, STREPTOMYCIN**).

See also:– atracurium, gallamine, pancuronium, suxamethonium.

TYRAMINE

As **EPHEDRINE** but more polar.

Present in certain foodstuffs esp. those prepared by fermentation with micro-organisms, e.g. cheeses & autolysed yeast products (Marmite, etc). Produced by decarboxylation of tyrosine.

Uses:– experimental tool only.

Precautions:– risk of severe hypertensive episode if tyramine- containing foods eaten by patients taking MAO-inhibitors.

See also:– dexamphetamine, ephedrine, phenylpropanolamine.

UNDECENOATES

Salts (usually zinc) of undecenoic acid (i.e. 11 carbon organic acid), which is a natural component of sweat and has antifungal properties.

Uses:– as topical antifungal agent (*Tinea*) – essentially superceded by the imidazole derivatives (see **MICONAZOLE**).

UREA

Excretion product for excess nitrogen. MW 60 – hence penetrates membranes via water filled pores.

Uses:– **i)** abortifacient – intra-amniotic injection causes placenta to degenerate
ii) osmotic diuretic
iii) as hydrating agent in skin creams.

Precautions:– concentration likely to rise excessively in patients with renal or hepatic failure; high blood concentrations induce confusion.

UROFOLLITROPHIN

See **FSH**.

UROKINASE

As **STREPTOKINASE**, but extracted from human urine.

VALPROATE

See **SODIUM VALPROATE.**

VASOPRESSIN

See **ADH.**

VERAPAMIL

Ca^{2+} channel blocker; inhibits Ca^{2+} movement through Ca^{2+} channels in vascular smooth muscle and through slow Ca^{2+} channels in cardiac tissue. Also delays inactivation of slow Ca^{2+} channels in cardiac cells and exhibits pronounced use-dependency.

Highly lipid soluble and rapidly metabolised by liver – hence "first-pass" effect after oral administration (ca. 80% metabolised).

Uses:– **i)** treatment of some kinds of supraventricular tachydysrhythmias (e.g. Wolff-Parkinson-White syndrome)
ii) prophylaxis of angina
iii) treatment of essential hypertension.

Precautions:– **i)** will exacerbate heart block
ii) likely to precipitate cardiac failure in patients taking antagonists at beta-adrenoceptors
iii) "first-pass" effect less marked in patients with liver failure.

See also:– nifedipine.

VERATRIDINE

Delays inactivation of Na^+ channel in nerve and muscle cells – hence hyperexcitability and repetitive firing. Possible mechanism is by displacing Ca^{2+} from membrane (effects attenuated if Ca^{2+} concentration raised).

One of the **VERATRUM ALKALOIDS**.

Uses:– experimental tool.

See also — batrachotoxin, dicophane.

VERATRUM ALKALOIDS

Group of alkaloids obtained from *Veratrum, Zygadenus and Schoenocaulon spp.* Pharmacological properties see **VERATRIDINE**.

VERCURONIUM

As d-TUBOCURARINE.

VINCA ALKALOIDS (VINCRISTINE & VINBLASTINE)

Inhibit spindle formation by disrupting microtubules and thereby arrest cell division in metaphase.

Poorly lipid soluble.

Natural source the Madagasca periwinkle plant (*Vinca rosea*).

Uses:– to treat malignant neoplastic disease:–
vincristine – acute leukaemias (esp. lymphoblastic), lymphomas
vinblastine – lymphomas & some solid tumours (e.g. testicular teratoma).

Precautions:– toxic effects are extension of normal pharmacology. Vincristine tends to be more neurotoxic than vinblastine.

VITAMIN K (PHYTOMENADIONE)

Essential cofactor for the production of blood clotting Factors VII, IX and X and prothrombin. Some comes from the diet, but most is absorbed from the GI tract where it is synthesised by the normal gut flora. The coumarin anticoagulants (e.g. **WARFARIN**) are vitamin K antagonists.

W

WARFARIN

Competitive inhibitor (close structural analogue) of **PHYTOMENADIONE** (vitamin K_1). Hence formation of prothrombin and Factors VII, IX and X. When existing supplies of these Factors are exhausted clotting ability is reduced (ca. 3 days).

Chemically a coumarin and very lipid soluble. Very highly protein-bound.

Uses:– i) oral anticoagulant in patients with deep vein thromboses, heart valve prostheses and in patients with non-pumping atria (e.g. uncontrolled atrial fibrillation) – prevents emboli
ii) as rodenticide.

Precautions:– i) induction of liver enzymes reduces blood concentration – hence bigger dose needed to maintain same anticoagulant effect. If exposure to inducing agent ceases dose will become an overdose and spontaneous bleeding will occur
ii) drugs with anticoagulant action additive (e.g. **ASPIRIN**)

iii) strain of "super rat" has evolved which is resistant to warfarin (in fact warfarin forms essential element of diet).

See also:– ancrod, dipyridamole, epoprostenol, heparin.

XANTHINE
Intermediate in neucleotide metabolism – precursor of uric acid.

See also:– allopurinol, methylxanthines.

XIPAMIDE
As **CHLORTHALIDONE.**

XYLOMETAZOLINE
As **METHOXAMINE.**

YEAST EXTRACT
Autolysed yeast, rich in vitamins, salt and cofactors. Also rich in amino acids and amines, especially **TYRAMINE** (decarboxylated tyrosine).

Precautions:– can precipitate hypertensive crisis in patients taking monoamine oxidase inhibitors.

YOHIMBINE
Competitive antagonist at α_2-adrenoceptors. Also local anaesthetic and antagonist at 5-HT receptors.

Chemically related to **RESERPINE** (but devoid of depleting activity).

Uses:– i) pharmacological tool
   ii) reputedly aphrodisiac.

ZIDOVUDINE

(Also known as azidothymidine or AZT). Thymidine analogue that inhibits replication in retrovirus infection, e.g. HIV (AIDS).

Uses:– palliative treatment of AIDS or AIDS-related complex.

Precautions:– interferes with normal pyrimidine metabolism – hence severe anaemia, neutropaenia and leukopenia, together with rashes and GI disturbance.

ZINC INSULIN

see **INSULIN**.

ZINC SULPHATE

Uses:– **i)** in creams and ointments for skin sores
ii) as zinc supplementation in zinc-deficiency, e.g. that accompanying protein calorie deficiency (Kwashiorkor)
iii) astringent in conjunctivitis.

ZUCLOPENTHIXOL

As **CHLORPROMAZINE**. Chemically a thioxanthine.

RAPID REFERENCE (ANTI-INDEX)

ADRENOCEPTORS & NORADRENERGIC NERVES

i) AGONISTS

a) Direct
ADRENALINE (α & β)
clonidine (α_2)
metaraminol (α)
methoxamine (α)
phenylephrine (α_1)
xylometazoline (α)
ISOPRENALINE (β)
dobutamine (β)
orciprenaline (β)
SALBUTAMOL (β_2)
fenoterol (β_2)
pirbuterol (β_2)
terbutaline (β_2)

b) Indirect
DEXAMPHETAMINE
diethylpropion
ephedrine
fencamfamin
methylphenidate
phenacetoperane
phenylpropanolamine
pipradol
tyramine

ii) PARTIAL AGONISTS
ergotamine (α)
acebutalol (β_1)
DCI (β)
pindolol (β)
practolol (β_1)

iii) ANTAGONISTS
PHENTOLAMINE (α)
PRAZOSIN (α_1)
chlorpromazine
indoramin (α_1)
yohimbine (α_2)
PHENOXYBENZAMINE (α; non-competitive)
dibenamine (α; non-competitive)
PROPRANOLOL (β)
nadolol (β)
oxprenolol (β)
sotalol (β)
timolol (β)
ATENOLOL (β_1)
labetalol (α & β)

iv) SYNTHESIS INHIBITORS
BENSERAZIDE
carbidopa
METHYLDOPA
METIROSINE

v) UPTAKE INHIBITORS
IMIPRAMINE (U_1)
amitryptyline (U_1)
cocaine (U_1)
desipramine (U_1)
methylphenidate (U_1)
mianserin (U_1)
nortryptyline (U_1)
phenacetoperane (U_1)
pipradol (U_1)
PHENOXYBENZAMINE (U_1 & U_2)

vi) COMT/MAO INHIBITORS
catechol (COMT)
PHENELZINE (MAO)
iproniazid (MAO)
isocarboxazid (MAO)
tranylcypromine (MAO)
SELEGILINE (MAO-B)

vii) NORADRENERGIC NEURONE BLOCKERS
GUANETHIDINE
bethanidine
bretylium
debrisoquine
RESERPINE
(TETRABENAZINE)

CHOLINOCEPTORS & CHOLINERGIC NERVES

i) AGONISTS
ACETYLCHOLINE (m,n)
benzoylcholine (m,n)
bethanechol (m_2)
carbachol (m,n)
furtrethonium (m)
McN-A-343 (m_1)
methacholine (m)
muscarine (m)
oxotremorine (m)
tremorine (m)
nicotine (n)
SUXAMETHONIUM (n skeletal muscle)
decamethonium (n skeletal muscle)
DMPP (n ganglia)
TMA (n ganglia)
deanol (choline precursor)

ii) PARTIAL AGONISTS
pilocarpine (m)

iii) ANTAGONISTS
ATROPINE (m)
benzhexol (m)
dicyclomine (m)
homatropine (m)
hyoscine (m)
ipatropium (m)
pirenzepine (m,)
tropicamide (m)
HEXAMETHONIUM (n ganglia)
mecamylamine (n ganglia)
pentolinium (n ganglia)
trimetaphan (n ganglia)
TEA (n ganglia)
d-TUBOCURARINE (n)
atracurium (n skeletal muscle)
gallamine (n skeletal muscle)
pancuronium (n skeletal muscle)
vercuronium (n skeletal muscle)
α-bungarotoxin (n skeletal muscle)

iv) RELEASE & SYNTHESIS INHIBITORS
BOTULINUS TOXIN
β-bungarotoxin
hemicholinium-3

v) FALSE TRANSMITTERS
acetyl triethylcholine (from triethyl choline)

vi) CHOLINESTERASE INHIBITORS
NEOSTIGMINE
edrophonium
physostigmine
ECOTHIOPATE (irreversible)
dyflos (irreversible)
PRALIDOXIME (reactivator)

INHIBITORS OF NEURONAL TRANSMISSION

i) LOCAL ANAESTHETICS (Na⁺ CHANNEL BLOCKERS)
LIGNOCAINE
amethocaine
benzocaine
bupivacaine
cinchocaine
prilocaine
procaine
saxitoxin
tetrodotoxin

ii) OTHER MECHANISMS
aconitine
batrachotoxin
dicophane
pyrethrin
veratridine

CNS TRANSMITTERS, etc.

i) DOPAMINE RECEPTORS & DOPAMINERGIC NERVES
a) AGONISTS
LEVODOPA (precursor)
BROMOCRYPTINE
amantidine
apomorphine
dobutamine
dopamine (transmitter)
DEXAMPHETAMINE (indirect)
amphonelic acid (indirect)
diethylpropion (indirect)
fencamfamin (indirect)

b) ANTAGONISTS
CHLORPROMAZINE
domperidone
droperidol
flupenthixol
haloperidol
metoclopramide
pimozide
spiperone
sulpiride
trifluoperazine
zuclopenthixol

c) DEPLETERS
RESERPINE
TETRABENAZINE

ii) GABA RECEPTORS & NERVES
a) AGONISTS
GABA
leptazol
picrotoxin

b) ANTAGONISTS
bicuculline

c) CATABOLISM INHIBITORS
amino-oxyacetic acid

iii) GLUTAMATE
a) AGONISTS
GLUTAMATE
kainic acid

iv) CNS/RESPIRATORY STIMULANTS/ CONVULSANTS
doxapram
leptazol
meclofenoxate
nikethimide
pemoline
picrotoxin
prolintane
STRYCHNINE

v) ENDORPHINS, etc.
  a) AGONISTS
    MORPHINE
    dextromoramide
    diamorphine
    diphenoxylate
    levorphanol
    methadone
    opium
    pethidine
    DEXTROMETHORPHAN
      (selective antitussive)
    dextrorphan (selective
      antitussive)
  b) PARTIAL AGONISTS
    buprenorphine
    codeine
    dihydrocodeine
    dextropropoxyphene
  c) ANTAGONISTS
    NALOXONE
  d) MIXED AGONISTS/
     ANTAGONISTS
    pentazocine

vi) ANXIOLYTICS/
    SEDATIVES/
    HYPNOTICS/ANTI-
    CONVULSANTS, etc.
  a) BENZODIAZEPINES
    DIAZEPAM
    chlordiazepoxide
    clonazepam
    flurazepam
    ketazolam
    lorazepam
    medazepam
    nitrazepam
    nordiazepam
    oxazepam
    temazepam
    triazolam
  b) BARBITURATES
    PHENOBARBITONE
    THIOPENTONE
    amylobarbitone
    butobarbitone
    pentobarbitone
    quinalbarbitone
  c) GENERAL
     ANAESTHETICS
    HALOTHANE
    chloroform
    cyclopropane
    diethyl ether
    enflurane
    methoxyflurane
    NITROUS OXIDE
    KETAMINE
    THIOPENTONE

  d) ANTI-CONVULSANTS
    DIAZEPAM
    PHENOBARBITONE
    PHENYTOIN
    carbamazepine
    ethosuximide
    sodium valproate
  e) OTHER
    ETHANOL
    CHLORAL HYDRATE
    chlormethiazole
    dichloralphenazone
    triclofos
    trichloroethanol (active
      metabolite)
    PARALDEHYDE
    DISULFIRAM (aldehyde
      dehydrogenase inhibitor)

vii) ANTI-DEPRESSANTS
  a) UPTAKE INHIBITORS
    IMIPRAMINE
    amitryptyline
    desipramine
    mianserin
  b) MAO INHIBITORS
    PHENELZINE
    iproniazid
    tranylcypromine
  c) MOOD STABILISERS
    LITHIUM

viii) HALLUCINOGENS
    LSD
    mescaline
    psilocin
    psilocybin

HEART

i) ANTI-DYSRHYTHMICS
    DIGOXIN
    ouabain
    LIGNOCAINE
    amiodarone
    phenytoin
    procainamide
    quinidine
    quinine
    VERAPAMIL

ii) INOTROPIC AGENTS
    DIGOXIN
    ouabain

iii) ANTI-ANGINAL AGENTS
    GLYCERYL TRINITRATE
    isosorbide dinitrate
    NIFEDIPINE
    nicardipine
    nitrendipine

PROPRANOLOL
ATENOLOL

ANTI-PARASITIC DRUGS
(including antibiotics, etc.)

i) ANTIBIOTICS, etc.
PENICILLIN
benzylpenicillin
amoxycillin
ampicillin
azlocillin
flucloxacillin
phenoxymethylpenicillin
ticarcillin
clavulinic acid (β-lactamase inhibitor)
probenecid (secretion inhibitor)
BLEOMYCIN
CEPHRADINE
cefuroxime
CHLORAMPHENICOL
clindamycin
COLISTIN
CYCLOSERINE
ERYTHROMYCIN
ETHAMBULOL
GENTAMICIN
kanamycin
neomycin
streptomycin
ISONIAZID
METRONIDAZOLE
RIFAMPICIN
SULPHAMETHIZOLE
dapsone
sulphamethoxazole
sulphapyridine
TETRACYCLINE
chlortetracycline
doxycycline
minocycline
oxytetracycline
dilanoxide furoate (amoebicide)
PRIMAQUINE (antimalarial)

ii) TRANSCRIPTION INHIBITORS
CHLOROQUINE (anti-malarial)
quinine (anti-malarial)
cycloheximide
doxorubicin

iii) ANTI-METABOLITES
METHOTREXATE
actinomycin D
azothioprine (prodrug of mercaptopurine)
cytarabine
fluorouracil
mercaptopurine
vinca alkaloids

iv) ALKYLATING AGENTS, etc.
CYCLOPHOSPHAMIDE
busulphan
chlorambucil
cisplatin
MESNA (acrolein ligand)

v) ANTI-VIRAL AGENTS
ACYCLOVIR
amantadine
zidovudine

vi) ANTI-FUNGAL AGENTS
benzoic acid
GRISEOFULVIN
MICONAZOLE
ketoconazole
NYSTATIN
amphotericin
tolnaftate
undecenoates

vii) INSECTICIDES, etc.
benzoyl benzoate
carbaryl
dicophane
monosulfiram
pyrethrin

viii) ANTI-ASCARIDS, etc.
bephenium
diethylcarbamazine

5-HT RECEPTORS, etc.

i) AGONISTS
5-HT (SEROTONIN)
fenfluramine (indirect)

ii) PARTIAL AGONISTS
METHYSERGIDE
metergoline
metitepine

iii) ANTAGONISTS
cinanserin
cyproheptadine
ketanserin
pizotifen

HISTAMINE RECEPTORS, etc.

i) AGONISTS
HISTAMINE (H_1 & H_2)
betahistine (H_1)
impromidine (H_1)
betazol (H_2)
dimaprit (H_2)

ii) ANTAGONISTS
CHLORPHENIRAMINE (H_1)
astemizole (H_1)
brompheniramine (H_1)
carbinoxamine (H_1)

chlorcyclizine (H$_1$)
cinnarizine (H$_1$)
cyclizine (H$_1$)
dimenhydrinate (H$_1$)
diphenhydramine (H$_1$)
hydroxyzine (H$_1$)
ketotifen (H$_1$)
meclozine (H$_1$)
mepyramine (H$_1$)
pizotifen (H$_1$)
promethazine (H$_1$)
terfenadine (H$_1$)
tripelennamine (H$_1$)
PHENOXYBENZAMINE (H$_1$;
    non-competitive)
CIMETIDINE (H$_2$)
ranitidine (H$_2$)

iii) RELEASE INHIBITORS
SODIUM CROMOGLYCATE
ketotifen

ANTI-PYRETIC ANALGESICS & NON-STEROIDAL ANTI-INFLAMMATORIES

i) MIXED ACTION
ASPIRIN
amidopyrine
azapropazone
benorylate
diflunisal
fenoprofen
flurbiprofen
ibuprofen
indomethacin
ketoprofen
meclofenamate
mefenamic acid
methyl salicylate
naproxen
oxyphenbutazone
phenazone
phenylbutazone
piroxicam
sulindac
tolmetin
SULPHASALAZINE
5-aminosalicylate (metabolite of
    SULPHASALAZINE)

ii) ANTI-PYRETIC ONLY
PARACETAMOL
phenacetin (prodrug of
    paracetamol)
ACETYLCYSTEINE (glutathione
    replenisher)
methionine (glutathione
    replenisher)

iii) OTHERS
ALLOPURINOL
colchicine
SODIUM AUROTHIOMALATE
auranofin
aurothioglucose
probenecid

PROSTANOIDS, etc.
arachidonic acid (precursor)
alprostadil (PGE$_1$)
dinoprost (PGF$_{2\alpha}$)
dinoprostone (PGE$_2$)
epoprostenol (prostacyclin)
leukotrienes
SRSa
thromboxanes

KININS
BRADYKININ
kallidin
kallikrein (enzyme)
aprotinin (proteolytic enzyme
    inhibitor)

BLOOD CLOTTING SYSTEM

i) ANTI-COAGULANTS
HEPARIN
WARFARIN
acenocoumarol
nicoumarol
ANCROD

ii) ANTIDOTES
PROTAMINE SULPHATE
VITAMIN K (PHYTOMENADIONE)

iii) CLOT PROMOTERS
AMINOCAPROIC ACID
tranexamic acid

iv) ANTI-PLATELET AGENTS
dipyridamole

v) THROMBOLYTICS
STREPTOKINASE
plasmin
urokinase

DIURETICS

i) POTASSIUM SPARING
AMILORIDE
triamterine

ii) THIAZIDES
BENDROFLUAZIDE
chlorthalidone
indapamide

xipamide

iii) HIGH CEILING
FRUSEMIDE
ethacrynic acid

iv) CARBONIC ANHYDRASE INHIBITORS
ACETAZOLAMIDE

ENDOCRINE SYSTEM

i) ADRENO-CORTICOIDS, etc.
FLUDROCORTISONE
PREDNISOLONE
aldosterone
beclomethasone
betamethasone
clobetasone
corticosterone
deoxycortone
dexamethasone
hydrocortisone
SPIRONOLACTONE (aldosterone antagonist)
androstenedione (precursor)
AMINOGLUTETHIMIDE (synthesis inhibitor)

ii) SEX HORMONES, etc.
dehydroepiandrosterone (sex steroid intermediate)
ETHINYLOESTRADIOL (oestrogen)
dienoestrol (oestrogen)
17-β-oestradiol (oestrogen)
quinoestrol (oestrogen)
stilboestrol (oestrogen)
CLOMIPHENE (oestrogen antagonist)
tamoxifen (oestrogen antagonist)
NORETHISTERONE (progestagen)
ethisterone (progestagen)
medroxyprogesterone (progestagen)
progesterone (progestagen)
TESTOSTERONE (androgen)
5-α-dihydrotestosterone (androgen)
nandrolone (androgen)
stanazolol (androgen)
CYPROTERONE (androgen antagonist)

iii) PITUITARY HORMONES, PEPTIDES, etc.
ADH (vasopressin)
desmopressin
felypressin
lypressin
terlipressin
OXYTOCIN
ergometrine
PROLACTIN (lactogen)
SOMATREM

growth hormone
somatostatin (GH release inhibitor)
angiotensin I
angiotensin II
saralasin (angiotensin antagonist)
CAPTOPRIL (ACE inhibitor)
enalapril (ACE inhibitor)
aprotinin (proteolytic enzyme inhibitor)

iv) THYROID/PARATHYROID
SALCATONIN
calcitonin
THYROXINE
iodine
CARBIMAZOLE (anti-thyroid)
methimazole (anti-thyroid)
potassium perchlorate (anti-thyroid)
propylthiouracil (anti-thyroid)

v) TROPHINS, etc.
ACTH
TETRACOSACTRIN
FSH
HCG
LH
menotrophin
PMHG
PMSG
DANAZOL (inhibits gonadotrophin release)

vi) ENDOCRINE PANCREAS
a) Parenteral Hypoglycaemic Agents
INSULIN

b) Oral Hypoglycaemic Agents
TOLBUTAMIDE
acetoheximide
chlorpropamide
glibenclamide
glicazide
glipizide
tolazamide
METFORMIN

c) OTHERS
alloxan (destroys B-cells)
glucagon

SMOOTH MUSCLE RELAXANTS

i) PHOSPHODIESTERASE INHIBITORS
THEOPHYLLINE
aminophylline
caffeine
choline theophyllinate
theobromine

ii) OTHERS
GLYCERYL TRINITRATE
isosorbide dinitrate
cromokalim
nicorandil
pinacidil
diazoxide
hydralazine
minoxidil
SODIUM NITROPRUSSIDE

GASTROINTESTINAL TRACT

i) STOMACH
CIMETIDINE
ranitidine
gastrin
pentagastrin
omeprazole

ii) LAXATIVES
bisacodyl
danthron
dioctyl sodium succinate
magnesium sulphate (Epsom salts)
methylcellulose

MISCELLANEOUS

i) K⁺ CHANNEL BLOCKERS
apamin
TEA

ii) K⁺ CHANNEL OPENERS
CROMOKALIM
nicorandil
pinacidil

iii) MUCOLYTICS
acetylcysteine
bromhexine
carbocisteine

iv) CALCIUM RELEASE INHIBITORS
dantrolene

v) CHELATING AGENTS
DESFERRIOXAMINE
dimercaprol
EDTA
EGTA
penicillamine

vi) SKIN
a) UV FILTERS
aminobenzoic acid
b) ANTI-PSORIATIC AGENTS
dithranol
c) KERATOLYTIC AGENTS
salicylic acid